Praise for *The Secret Wisdom of a Woman's Body*

"There are gifts of insight and awareness in this book for women of all ages."
—Connie Goldman, former National Public Radio reporter
and author of *The Ageless Spirit*

"Pat Samples offers women in the second half of life a powerful opportunity to explore their complex relationships to their bodies and their deepest selves."
—Evelyn Torton Beck, PhD,
Professor Emerita of Women's Studies, University of Maryland

"This is a must read for women of all ages who dare to face the cultural myths about women's bodies."
—Marilyn J. Mason, PhD, psychologist and former faculty,
University of Minnesota Medical School Program in Human Sexuality,
and the author of *Seven Mountains: Life Lessons from a Climber's Journal*

"With wisdom and grace, Pat Samples offers us accessible, intriguing exercises which open us to the possibility of truly appreciating and actually celebrating our aging bodies. If you want to be inspired, read this!"
—Karen Roeper, founder and director of Essential Motion

"As a somatic teacher and healer, I find Pat Samples' book to be a wonderful, practical, easy-to-read, and user-friendly tool for women looking to embrace their body."
—Debbie Rosas, co-founder of the Nia Technique, Inc.

"A must-read for any woman who is ready to reclaim the beauty and wisdom that comes from cherishing our body just the way it is. This is a welcome antidote to an ageist culture that glorifies youth and skinny bodies. At last we can step back into our power."
—Dr. Karen Wolfe, physician and author of
Create the Body Your Soul Desires

About the Author

Pat Samples, MFA, MA, is a writer and transformational educator who helps people tap into their inner wisdom and creativity as they age. She is the author of nine other books, including *Body Odyssey: Lessons from the Bones and Belly* and *Daily Comforts for Caregivers*. Samples has given hundreds of talks and workshops internationally on conscious aging, body wisdom, caregiving, spirituality, creative writing, and inspired living.

In her writing, speaking, and teaching, she draws on a diverse background in health care, social services, ministry, and the arts. Samples has an MA in human development and an MFA in creative writing. She is one of the founders and leaders of the Minnesota Creative Arts and Aging Network and is also active in the work of the National Center for Creative Aging and the American Society on Aging. Samples was the director of an inner-city arts education program and theatre for nine years. She lives in a Minneapolis suburb, where she enjoys walking, biking, dancing, and spiritual conversations with her friends. Please visit her website at www.patsamples.com.

To Write to the Author

If you wish to contact the author or would like more information about this book, please write to the author in care of Llewellyn Worldwide and we will forward your request. Both the author and publisher appreciate hearing from you and learning of your enjoyment of this book and how it has helped you. Llewellyn Worldwide cannot guarantee that every letter written to the author can be answered, but all will be forwarded. Please write to:

Pat Samples
℅ Llewellyn Worldwide
2143 Wooddale Drive, Dept. 978-0-7387-1159-1
Woodbury, MN 55125-2989, U. S. A.

Please enclose a self-addressed stamped envelope for reply,
or $1.00 to cover costs. If outside the USA, enclose an
international postal reply coupon.

Many of Llewellyn's authors have websites with additional information and resources. For more information, please visit our website at www.llewellyn.com.

Pat Samples

The Secret
Wisdom
of a
Woman's
Body

Freeing Yourself to
Live Passionately
and *Age Fearlessly*

Llewellyn Publications
Woodbury, Minnesota

First Edition
First Printing, 2007

Book design by Steffani Sawyer
Editing by Brett Fechheimer
Cover art © 2007 by Image Source/Superstock
Cover design by Ellen Dahl

Llewellyn is a registered trademark of Llewellyn Worldwide, Ltd.

Library of Congress Cataloging-in-Publication Data for *The Secret Wisdom of a Woman's
Body* is on file at the Library of Congress.
ISBN: 978-0-7387-1159-1

Llewellyn Worldwide does not participate in, endorse, or have any authority or responsibility concerning private business transactions between our authors and the public.
   All mail addressed to the author is forwarded but the publisher cannot, unless specifically
instructed by the author, give out an address or phone number.
   Any Internet references contained in this work are current at publication time, but the
publisher cannot guarantee that a specific location will continue to be maintained. Please
refer to the publisher's website for links to authors' websites and other sources.
   Cover model used for illustrative purposes only and may not endorse or represent the
book's subject.

Llewellyn Publications
A Division of Llewellyn Worldwide, Ltd.
2143 Wooddale Drive, Dept. 978-0-7387-1159-1
Woodbury, Minnesota 55125-2989, U.S.A.
www.llewellyn.com

Printed in the United States of America

Contents

Acknowledgments

Splendid teachers have introduced me to the wisdom of our bodies. My gratitude to Cherie McCoy, Brian Brooks, Manfred Fischbeck, and Karen Roeper is immeasurable. I also owe a substantial debt to Thomas Wright, co-creator of the Writing Your Own Permission Slip course, from which some of this book's examples are drawn.

Thanks to the members of the Free Motion group I lead each week, who romp with me as we explore and delight in the body's creativity. Every week dancing with them takes me to a state of awe.

Thanks also to my women's group who have believed in me and my work and who have honored the stories my body needed to tell. Anne Boever and Marjorie Spagl have waded through deep waters with me over the years, and I love them dearly.

Other cherished friends and encouragers while I worked on this book have been Rita Mays, Kathy Olson, Joy Anderson, Ron Nelsen, Cynthia Ryden Austin, Julia Jergensen-Edelman, Sheila Asato, Jeff Sylvestre, and Mary Lange. They listened to me, cheered me on, and sometimes gave me just the right idea when I needed it. Friends make all the difference. Thank you. I also appreciate the immensely helpful feedback from early readers of the manuscript: Terri Burks, Sheila Rubin, and Evelyn Torton Beck, as well as members of my writers group.

Many artists and advocates with a passion for vital and creative aging have inspired my own work in aging. Among those whose leadership and personal encouragement have been a lighthouse for me are Susan Perlstein, Sally Hebson, Peggy Thompson, Jan Hively, Connie Goldman, Evelyn Fairbanks, Priscilla Herbison, Gene Cohen, and Maria Genné.

After acquisitions editor Carrie Obry approached me about doing a book for Llewellyn, she was a wizard at drawing out my best ideas and then guiding me in how to sift out the chaff from the manuscript's first draft. Production editor Brett Fechheimer's gentle manner and skilled attention to accuracy and clarity made me at ease with the editing process. I appreciate being supported with such competence. Thank you also to all the people who have allowed me to tell their stories within these pages.

Other books written or co-authored by Pat Samples

Body Odyssey: Lessons from the Bones and Belly
Daily Comforts for Caregivers
Self-Care for Caregivers: A Twelve Step Approach
Comfort and Be Comforted: Reflections for Caregivers
With Open Arms
The Twelve Steps and Dual Disorders
The Twelve Steps and Dual Disorders Workbook
Older Adults in Treatment
Older Adults after Treatment

Introduction

"Every life has stories mistold, stories approached watch-
fully, stories never finished, and truth of its own, hidden
even from ourselves."

LINDA HOGAN, *The Woman Who Watches Over the World*

"You store power in your body... If you ignore the signals
your body sends to you, you will begin to dissipate your
power and begin to destroy your body through stress, because
you are not paying attention to who you really are."

LYNN ANDREWS, *The Writing Spirit*

Some women love their bodies; some hate them. I'm in the love-my-body camp. Well, maybe not every single minute. Sometimes I feel pretty awkward and uncomfortable in my body. Though I'm satisfied with how I look, generally speaking, I'm not thrilled with my blotchy skin and extra-thin hair. I'm in decent shape, but the list of supplements I'm taking for this and that is growing, even though I work out, eat organic foods, and follow the tips I read on women's health.

Like most women in their middle and older years, I don't like the idea of my body going south. Yet most of the time I enjoy living in my body—a lot. Here's why: thanks to all the experiences I've been through in over six decades of life, my body has become a treasure chest full of emotional and spiritual wisdom just waiting to be discovered. I've found that the secrets my body is literally aching to tell me every day can be great sources of delight, healing, and creativity if I'm willing to pay attention. My body has become a much-valued friend and teacher, constantly revealing clues to the mysteries of my life.

Your body, too, is a treasure chest—a rich archive of your life experiences with secrets aplenty to tell you. Discovering these secrets will enrich your life and ease your passage through midlife and beyond. This book offers a guide to unveiling the secrets hiding in your body.

Years of personal and professional curiosity led me to this discovery about the wisdom hiding in the body of every woman. Around the time of my fiftieth birthday, I knew I'd turned a major corner in my life. Another fifty years or more lay ahead, or at least that was a possibility. This realization both excited and scared me. I wondered how I could make the most of my remaining years. I'd gotten to fifty with some degree of success—a career as a writer and international speaker, a good circle of friends, and a son I was proud of. I'd survived a divorce, financial stresses, and plenty of other hurdles, and I finally felt like a grown-up. Now I faced this new thrilling, yet daunting, horizon. I wasn't too interested in thinking about retirement yet, but I did want to create the second half of my life in such a way that I didn't end up with bingo games or endless golfing as my ultimate destiny. I wanted to shape my next fifty years with meaning and purpose, and I wanted to have a good time doing it. My mind was curious. My spirit was eager. I was raring to go. But what about my body? Would it hold up for the duration, or would I be sagging and dragging my way through the coming years? Would I like how I looked and felt?

Not that I had any major health issues at that point. Yet shoulder and elbow pains from years of bad-form tennis serves had taken me off the courts and made lifting grocery bags and working at the computer more difficult. Hot flashes, wrinkle lines on my face, and spots appearing in my vision revealed signs of "aging." Increasingly, numerous body stresses from an overly busy life and from lingering emotional residue were sending me to see doctors and healers of all sorts. Besides that, anti-aging campaigns blared at me everywhere, reinforcing my concerns by telling me I had to take drastic—and even plastic—steps if I didn't want to look and feel old. None of these approaches to the aging body inspired me. Something else was needed if I were going to find confidence and ease in my body through my middle years and beyond.

I decided it was time to get to know my body in a new way—intimately. Since it was "talking" to me more and more, I was going to become its student. I was curious to know: what would I learn if listened *deeply?*

About that time I began teaching a course called "Writing Your Own Permission Slip." In it, I invited students to playfully and reflectively pay attention to the lifetime of stories living in their bones and bellies—and to write and revise these stories in ways that would empower and free them. To develop the class, I drew on my years of involvement in theatre and the other creative arts, my longtime study and teaching work in spiritual and emotional growth, and my growing interest in the wisdom of the human body. I used music, imagery, dramatic improvisation, and a variety of body awareness processes to prepare the students for writing exercises. As I've continued to teach this class over the years, I've witnessed remarkable transformations emerging from these simple activities. I have listened as women who wanted to sing found their voices. I have watched as women who were overtired and uninspired found the power to say no, or broke loose into the freedom of play. I have celebrated with women who wanted to go to Africa or grad school, or who wanted to move past mourning as they claimed the freedom deep inside themselves to say yes.

The class has also fostered my own process of learning about body wisdom because I complete all the class activities and assignments myself. I've learned to pay attention to how fast I'm walking throughout my day, and to slow that pace to match my internal rhythms instead of external clock demands. I've discovered how to declare my intentions for my life not just as a mental exercise but in a fully embodied way. I have discovered how my body can guide me to find what I call the Spirit or the God-life within me, so I can enjoy and express the gifts of the soul. More and more, because of this class and because of other body awareness studies and teaching I have done, I feel at home in my body. I've come to honor its ways of knowing and its desires.

Many teachers and guides have helped me as I've learned to draw upon my somatic resources. One of my strongest and most unusual lessons came in a workshop I attended in my mid-fifties. It was led by Karen Roeper, a Zen-like former dancer and the founder of an international program in body awareness called Essential Motion. I had been suffering from neck tension for a long time, and it had worsened over the years. Women's bodies are smart like that. They signal with increasing urgency that we have a problem until it hurts enough to get our attention. The older we get, the more persistent the body becomes at asking us to look at what's wrong and fix it. I asked Roeper for help in getting to the bottom of my persistent neck tension.

My strategy had always been to try *relaxing* the tension, but Roeper invited me to let it be. In fact, she encouraged me to pay close attention to the tension without trying to change it, yet to be alert to any changes that might occur. With her calm guidance, I quieted my mind and became a curious student of my body, open to what it wanted me to know. Almost as if my body understood it had my full attention, it went all out to let me in on its surprising emotional content. Slowly, the tension in my neck grew. It spread up into my jaw and down into my arms, shoulders, and torso. The movement was so intense and extreme that I felt as if someone else had taken over my body parts, moving me like a muscled marionette, but from the inside rather than with strings. As Roeper encouraged me to stay with this strange pressure-cooker intensity, my body contorted into what felt like a grotesque form—with my head bent backward, my arms extended behind me, and my hands facing toward the wall behind me in a pushing position. My whole body felt as if I were pushing backwards against the wall, while at the same time pushing forward with my torso. Even my facial muscles tightened fiercely to manage this extreme double effort.

When the pushing sensations became painfully intense, Roeper asked me with genuine interest, "What are you pushing, Pat?"

In my book *Body Odyssey: Lessons from the Bones and Belly*, I describe how I responded and what happened next:

....

"Nothing," I answered. A vast stillness followed. Almost at once, the accumulated pressure began to dissipate.

I stood there, quietly stunned, taking in fully the absurdity of what I'd been experiencing—pushing when there was nothing to be pushed. It was so familiar, this making of my life a struggle, everything taking enormous effort. I had lived that way for years—for all the years my neck had been complaining. I'd do things like shopping for a new car when exhausted, on a below-zero day, rather than waiting for better conditions. Driving long hours on trips without stopping—having to "push on." Trying endlessly to make a marriage work that just wouldn't.

"Maybe there is nothing to push," she responded quietly, echoing my words but amplifying their meaning. My whole musculature had already begun to

register this very notion. The painful pushing sensations rapidly subsided. Tension dropped away. I felt myself standing taller. I was not pushing.

....

In this incident, I became profoundly aware of the remarkable wisdom living in my body—in *all* women's bodies. I realized how eloquently our body lets us in on its secrets—the secrets we keep from ourselves—when we become open to hearing those secrets. In my case, I discovered how much I had been trying to *push* my way through life. I recognized how faithfully my body had been trying to tell me for years that constantly pushing was a painful and difficult way to live.

Once my tension dropped away, I felt a new sense of freedom. Roeper had me walk around the room to experience this new feeling of "not pushing." The results were comical. At first, I could barely walk. My body had been trained since childhood for dedicated, perfectionistic hard work. Now I was awkwardly relearning how to move around in a freed-up body, to just "hang out." Before long, as I felt myself gliding across the room with ease, I was almost giddy.

The new confidence and freedom I felt in my whole being from learning how to stop pushing and "hang out" evoked a deep sense of awe and respect for my body. This remarkable experience was one of many I've had that have helped me become an avid student and appreciator of my body. I also pursued a master's degree in human development, with an emphasis on conscious aging and body wisdom. I read voraciously and studied with master teachers in body awareness, mind-body-spirit integration, and the arts. I also talked with many, many women—mothers in midlife stressed by their multiple responsibilities of parenting teenagers while working full-time and undertaking community involvement; women seeking help from the medical and alternative healthcare systems in ways that honor the mind-body-spirit connection; women turning forty or fifty or sixty who want to feel "young" but who don't want to play the "I'm only thirty-nine" game; women who have survived illness and abuse and deception, and who want to heal and make meaning from their experiences; and so many more. Most importantly, I listened deeply to my own body.

I pursued all this study because I wanted to make sense of the changes and distress signals in my body that seemed to increase over the years. I wanted a practical approach to living peacefully and confidently in my body as it got older, even as the culture around me finds fault with aging bodies and glorifies youth. I searched for simple ways of understanding and learning from my body that don't require complicated sets of practices or a set of lingo to remember. And I wanted to learn these things not only for myself but also to share with other women who have the same desires.

From all these experiences has emerged my fervent commitment to change how our culture views the aging body—and especially to change how we women feel about and experience our own bodies. With a little guidance and support, I'm convinced that each of us can uncover the emotional brilliance in our body as we move through midlife and into our later years. We can express ourselves confidently and creatively, and live from our spiritual essence. Every woman can experience her body as a vibrant, creative force. We can have the sense of freedom that comes, in part, from feeling at home in our own body.

Learn to tap your body's riches

My curiosity and my commitment have led me to discover and develop many simple approaches to achieving these goals. Some of them I describe in *Body Odyssey*, a memoir and guide I wrote to celebrate and demonstrate the emotional and spiritual wisdom that women's bodies accumulate over the years. Since I wrote that book, I've developed many more ways of accessing the body's wealth of wisdom. I've shared these approaches with thousands of women in classes and workshops I've led across North America—as well as through my books, articles, newsletters, and websites. In this book, I'm sharing them with you.

This book is a guide for women in midlife and older who are hungry for more meaning, better health, and more confidence and vibrancy in their lives (though many of its lessons apply to women of all ages and to men as well). I wrote it to help you tap into the treasury of your body. I want to help you regain the childlike sense of marvel and curiosity you once had about your body, if you've lost it. I want you to be able to feel your aliveness and to heal what hurts.

Your body is an evocative storyteller and teacher. It contains volumes of your history, with all its intrigue, humor, and angst. The collection of stories expands with each passing day. The older you are, the more stories you'll have to draw from and the more likely the long-buried ones will emerge unbidden, often showing up as pain or tensions or urges. I invite you to "read" these stories, enjoy them, learn from them. What could be more fascinating than the saga of your own life that's been imprinted in your bones and belly!

You might wonder: how can I do this? How can I "read" or "listen to" my body? Where do I begin? Even once you start this curious exploration, you may find your body's "language" unfamiliar and wonder how to understand what you find as you turn page after page. Why is my head hurting? What is this pain in my neck? Rest assured that learning to read your body will be like returning home. It may take a while, but as with a hungry baby seeking its mother's breast, your natural instincts will be refreshed once you learn to trust them again.

One woman, Kathy Shea, describes this refresher effect after she was introduced to the ideas and activities offered in this book: "I've been relating differently to my body since. All it took was the reminder that they're all alive, these body parts, and that they deserve to be honored and appreciated—however old we might be. I even notice an affectionate, chummy feeling toward my body that could lead to fond acceptance of change over time. I also notice a new intimacy, stemming from the idea that my body can tell me important things if I notice, that it's my advance team."

Your body will indeed be your advance team, your ally showing you the way. This book will help you learn how to follow its lead. Reading these pages and doing the suggested activities won't stop you from aging, but doing so will give you a way to experience what happens in your body with a fresh sense of wonder and purpose. You may even find relief from physical symptoms. You will surely find a greater understanding of why you hurt and what your body's promptings mean.

You can also find many knowledgeable and caring people to assist you in learning the body's wise ways. Bodyworkers, spiritual teachers, energy healers, personal coaches, performing artists, or other guides may help you gain greater access to your body's revelations. If some of what you discover seems too painful to manage by yourself, it's especially important to seek the counsel of a therapist or other professional who has expertise in dealing with body trauma.

Stories are often the best teachers, and you will find many of them in these pages. These are true stories from my life and from the lives of other women I've met. A few of the stories are composites of experiences I've heard from more than one woman. In most cases, the identities of the people in the stories have been disguised to protect their privacy. You'll also find many activities and exercises in these pages that will help you try out these approaches to body wisdom for yourself.

How to use this book

The book has three parts. If you're new to exploring the wisdom of the body, part 1 of this book, entitled "Wake Up to Your Body," will give you the basics. It will show you how to make friends with your body, cherish it, listen to it, and enjoy it in ways you've never dreamed of (or maybe you have!). If you're already quite at home in your body—perhaps because you do yoga, breathwork, or mindfulness practices—you may want to skip right to part 2. In part 2, "Heal Your Body," you'll find many stories and practical ideas that can help you heal from emotional, physical, and spiritual pain. Part 3, "Create with Abandon," invites you to play and express yourself in artistic and other creative ways. You'll also learn how to access the spiritual well from which your creativity flows.

Some of the processes and activities I suggest work best when done with at least one other person. Consider inviting a friend or a group you regularly meet with to join you in this exploratory process. You can even form your own small group of women, and help each other to discover the stories in your body that are waiting to be told.

But you don't need anyone else to get the benefits of this book. Most of the activities you can do on your own. You'll have lots of them to choose from. At the end of each chapter, I present you with three sets of activities. "Observe and Reflect" activities help you notice your bodily experiences in new ways and to look for their lessons. Then I suggest "Write" activities that you can do in your journal. A third set of activities, called "Live," helps you implement the chapter ideas into your day-to-day life.

The exercises will make it easier for you to find the wisdom that your body holds. I use many of them myself and teach them in classes and workshops. Try them. Have fun with them. Change them to suit your personal style. Give yourself permission to do something you've never tried before or haven't done in a long time. Make up some body-learning activities of your own. Let your body and your mind have a field day.

Enjoy the rewards

Enormous rewards await you when you attend to what your body has to say. Through mindful and playful attention to your body's stories past and present, you'll learn core emotional and spiritual lessons that will foster authentic, integrated living. You'll find meaning from what you've been through, and you'll more easily be able to resolve lingering, painful issues. As you come to feel more and more at home in your body, you'll find a renewed sense of passion, aliveness, and creativity. You'll recognize your body as an invaluable resource and guide right up until your last breath. You may even shed your fear of aging. Get ready for a fascinating journey into your own somatic mysteries.

Part 1

Wake Up to Your Body

"I began to feel my body in a way that was new to me. It was like listening to an old friend that I cared about."

CHERI CLAMPETT, "A Knowing Beyond Words," *Wisdom of the East*

What Are These Things Dangling at the Ends of My Arms?

Every Friday morning, I gather with a group of women in their mid-forties and older for a creative dance session called Free Motion. Guided only by my occasional prompts and ethereal melodies from a CD, we all swirl, sway, bend, roll, and tumble wordlessly in our own way, luxuriating in the pleasure of our bodies moving freely. The experience is meditative and playful, relaxing and refreshing. When we're finished, we sit silently in a circle, still in a somewhat dreamlike state after slipping away from our thoughts and letting ourselves *be moved* by our bodies. We try to put into words something of what has happened for us.

Recently, Cecilia—a newcomer with long, stringy gray hair and a deeply wrinkled smile—spoke slowly into the silence: "Right from the beginning, when we were just lying there on the floor and starting to move, I thought to myself: *where* have I *been?!*" She added, "Everything in me kind of shook loose." It was as if she had left home for a long time and finally found her way back—to her body, to the home of her spirit. After a moment of quiet, she sighed deeply and continued, "We're so busy all the time doing so many things that seem so important, and they aren't really that important."

Most of us are getting smarter about our bodies as we age. To stay fit, we've learned how to strengthen core muscles and walk or bike for cardio benefits. We rely on mammograms and MRIs to detect abnormalities. We surf the Web for information about how our parts work, how to keep them tuned up, and how to fix or manage them when they're not. But acquiring information and following wellness guidelines are not the same as knowing our body from the inside out—*being* in our body, *living* in it. For Cecilia, allowing her body to move freely, according to her inner impulses, brought her back to living in her body—and gave her access to its priceless wisdom.

Pay attention

What does it mean to live in your body? How does it feel? How do you know you're alive?

Knowing starts with the simple act of paying attention. We routinely pay attention to our body in certain ways every day. We bathe, fix our hair, and trim our nails to keep our body clean and looking attractive. We eat to stave off hunger, ideally eating what is nourishing. Many of us exercise to keep in shape, and we schedule a massage now and then. We may take medications and supplements or follow other procedures to deal with specific health problems. So far, so good. That covers basic body care and maintenance—even some all-important self-nurturing activities.

But how *alive* do we feel as we go through these experiences? How *conscious* are we? How *present* are we?

Check this out for yourself. Do you hurriedly grab a bite to eat? Do you use the speakerphone so you can set up an appointment or share gossip while brushing your hair and putting on your makeup? Are you rushing through your body care as a necessary chore so you can get on to other things? Or are you fully, consciously, lovingly present when you're tending to your body? If you're like many people, you may give your body only passing attention when you're taking care of it. And during the rest of the day, you may barely be aware of living in your body at all. What about right now? Notice your experience of your body at this moment. Are you "in" your body as you read this book? Or are you completely unaware of your sensations, your urges, your vitality?

Your body is worthy of your attention because it's the precious home for your spirit. It's how you experience being alive. It's your avenue for taking in your world and expressing yourself. Thomas Moore, in *Care of the Soul,* describes the human body as "the soul presented in its richest and most expressive form."

Too often, we're hardly "in" our body at all. Our attention is wrapped up in our thoughts. Many of us tend to be compulsive thinkers. Our mind is in charge. If our body is doing anything, it's acting in response to our thoughts. When our body doesn't perform according to expectation, it's common practice to give it a push with caffeine, exhaust it and make it ill with an overdose of activity, or pacify it with alcohol or pills or the promise of a golf game or yoga class soon.

What's happening in your body right now? Stop reading for a moment and observe. Feel your feet. Notice what your breath is doing. Observe any effort you're making in your jaw and facial muscles, your neck and shoulders—anywhere in your body. Notice what feels pleasurable. Be in your body. Give your attention to the physical experience of being alive.

As you continue reading this book, make a point to stop and do this body-awareness activity at least once during each chapter. You may find you'll want to do it periodically throughout your day. The more you practice being consciously present in your body, the more you'll feel like you're coming home.

Feel your body from the inside out

Some years ago, I became acquainted with the Subtle Self Work of Judith Blackstone, who teaches the practice of conscious living. I remember the first time I listened to one of her recorded tapes and heard this instruction: "Feel the space *inside* your arms. Feel what it's like to be live *inside* your arms." I was intrigued by this suggestion and directed my attention to that "space" inside my arms. As I did, I was surprised by the expanded internal sensation I felt within my arms, almost as if someone had pumped air into them. They felt larger than usual, as if more of me were there somehow. I sensed my arms not as appendages of a certain size and weight but as buoyant fields of energy, pulsing with life. My arms seemed to be floating and almost boundary-less. It was a giddy experience.

I used to play this particular tape whenever I had a panic attack, a problem I experienced for many years. These attacks always came on suddenly.

For little or no reason I could identify, I'd feel as if I'd nearly been hit by a truck. My heart rate would speed up. I'd feel dizzy, irritable, and short of breath. My thoughts would race and I'd become extremely fearful. This flood of physical and emotional responses sometimes continued for hours at a time. If I couldn't calm the panic readily, I would listen to Blackstone's tape.

After a few minutes of listening to her instructions and performing the activities she suggested, the attack would subside somewhat. When I got to the "feel the space inside your arms" activity, which was near the end of the tape, the panic would dissipate notably. The tape concluded with further guidance, inviting me to experience living "inside my body all at once." That cinched the panic relief. Now my whole body experienced an expanded, energized, yet calm, state. The frantic thoughts, rapid heartbeat, and overall agitated state of mind that had been with me when I started the tape were now gone. I was indeed living "inside" my body instead of in a state of fear about the future. I was living in the *now*.

The spiritual teacher Eckhart Tolle, best known for his book *The Power of Now*, devotes a whole chapter of that book to a similar notion of experiencing what he calls the "inner body." He also talks about it in *A New Earth: Awakening to Your Life's Purpose*, in which he writes: "Your inner body is not solid but spacious. It is . . . the life that animates the physical form." Tolle believes we can feel this spacious sense of the life within us by cultivating awareness of the inner body. "When waiting, when listening to someone, when pausing to look at the sky, a tree, a flower, your partner, or child, feel the aliveness within at the same time." When you are conscious of your body, aware of both its form and its formless animating force, says Tolle, you are living *here, now*, in the *present*.

As an infant, your mind was not occupied with thoughts. Your life was an all-body experience. You were feeling, smelling, hearing, moving. You were fully alive. Some of that experience of aliveness may have been lost as you grew up and learned to subdue the body in service to your mind and the authority figures around you. You may have come to feel distant from your body and its pleasures and wisdom. It's possible for you to regain the sense of fully living in your body, of being fully *here*. The exercise below will help get you started. It will allow you to acquaint yourself newly with your body through conscious attention. It will help you *know* what it means to feel alive in each area of your body. Test it for yourself. Discover what it feels like to be fully conscious of the experience of living in your body.

EXERCISE: CONSCIOUS BODY AWARENESS

Choose a time when you can give undivided attention to your body for fifteen minutes. Sit in a quiet place where you won't be disturbed. Close your eyes. Take several full breaths, noticing your belly rise and fall as you inhale and exhale. Observe the swirl of thoughts in your mind, and let it settle the way dust settles to the ground after the wind stills. With each breath, let your thoughts become quieter and quieter.

Bring your attention to your feet. Notice their weight. Notice where this weight feels heaviest—on the balls of your feet, the heels, the arches, or somewhere else. Pay attention to which parts of your feet touch the surface on which they're resting. What is the feeling where they touch this surface? No need to name this feeling. No need to think about it. Just experience *with awareness* the feeling of your feet touching what they are touching. Observe whether one foot feels different from the other. Be aware of other sensations in your feet. Is there any tingling anywhere? Tightness? Pain? Don't try to change anything. Just notice your experience with loving attention. Feel yourself living inside your feet. If it helps you to wiggle your toes and move your feet in order to feel their aliveness, you can do so, but do it slowly and with conscious attention.

Let your attention shift to your ankles and calves. Enjoy the experience of getting to know your ankles and calves from the inside out. Pay attention to the sensations that tell you their size, shape, and weight. Where do they hurt or feel restricted? Where do they feel vibrant, pulsing, alive? Feel yourself living inside your ankles and calves.

Become aware of your knees and thighs. Let yourself feel the life flowing through these areas of your body. Notice how your thighs feel as they press against the surface beneath them. Notice any temperature difference between the front and back of your thighs and between one thigh and the other. Feel your skin as it covers your thighs and surrounds your kneecaps.

See if you can sense the size of the space that your knees and thighs take up. Concentrate on sensing this physically from the inside rather than pursuing a *thought* about measurement. Move your legs a little, slowly, to give you even more of a sense of the aliveness of your body below your pelvis. As you do, notice which muscles tighten and loosen to allow this movement. Be aware of any discomfort you feel, and then expand your awareness to take in areas of your legs beyond the discomfort. Experience living inside the entire area of your legs and feet.

Bring your attention to your hips and pelvis. Become aware of the area at the floor of your pelvis. Notice any thoughts that may arise about putting your attention on this area, and let them drift by like clouds. Breathe easily and fully. Check for any movement in the lower part of your pelvis as you breathe. Feel the size and shape of this area. Notice any tension and observe any changes that take place as you bring your attention here. Feel your aliveness in this area. Expand your awareness to include all of your hips. Feel the pressure of your hips against the surface on which they rest. Notice any movement in your hip muscles as you breathe. Feel how much space your hips take up. Let any thoughts of judgment pass by in the wind. Just feel your sense of yourself in your hips taking up whatever space they take up. Bring your attention to your tailbone, sensing where it's located within the pelvic area. Notice any tension in the area around your tailbone and in your lower back. Breathe into that area and feel the movement of your tailbone and lower spine.

Shift your attention forward and upward to the area of your belly. Let your belly experience your breathing, and notice the movement that corresponds with each inhalation and exhalation. Feel how much space your belly takes up, again dismissing any thoughts of judgment. Just sense the feeling of being alive inside your belly. To the degree you're able, distinguish the particular feeling inside each organ within your belly. Let your curiosity guide you to notice how one area within your belly may feel different than another. Observe any activity or discomfort, any difference in temperature, any sense of emptiness or fullness.

Bring your attention to your upper torso. Notice your breathing and the rising and falling of your chest. Feel the movement of your ribs in the front and the back of your chest. Notice the rhythm of your breath. Feel the full size and shape of your chest as it expands. Feel the space inside your chest. Give your attention to your heart. See if you can feel the life within your heart. Feel your heartbeat. Notice any sense of discomfort or pleasure around your heart. Feel the energy that is moving through this area of your body.

Move your attention to your spine. Notice how it moves as you breathe. Starting with your tailbone, let your attention move slowly up your spine to the base of your skull, one vertebra at a time. As you repeat this activity over time, you will be able to notice each vertebra more distinctly. Be aware of the energy moving through your spine. Feel yourself living inside your spine. Feel your spine supporting your torso and your head.

Let your attention move to your head. Feel the size and weight of it atop your spine. Notice your face and, without touching it, feel its shape. Feel inside the skin and muscles that cover your face and your entire skull. Feel inside your eyes, inside your mouth, inside your tongue. Notice whether your jaw is relaxed or not. Feel inside your brain, both sides of it. Feel your whole sense of yourself inside your head.

Become aware of your shoulders. Breathe into them. Notice their rising and falling. Feel yourself getting taller as you breathe into this area. Be aware of the shape of your shoulders—and any sensation of holding that you're experiencing there. Is one shoulder higher than the other? There's nothing you need to change as you observe these areas of your body. Just let yourself be curious. Notice the muscle tension that keeps your head upright and any tension that causes discomfort. Observe any changes that happen as you focus attention on your shoulders.

Notice how your shoulders connect with your arms. Feel the weight of your arms hanging at your sides. Experience any differences between your two arms. Does one feel more inclined to action? Notice any tension or pain. Feel the sensation of your arms touching whatever they're touching. Let your breath move through your arms, and feel the space inside your arms. Wiggle them slightly if it helps you experience your arms as being alive, as being *you*.

With your attention now dropping to your hands, experience your hands as part of your arms. Feel the energy moving through your arms and hands, into your fingers. Notice what it feels like to be alive inside your hands, inside each of your fingers. Feel your hands in a state of rest. Observe any differences between them. Wiggle your hands a little, noticing where that movement originates and what is happening inside your hands as you move them. Feel the relationship of your hands to the rest of your body.

Let your attention now expand to include your entire body. Breathe into your whole body and let your body expand to its full size. Your body is made up mostly of space. Feel the space inside your body. Experience life flowing through this space, through your body. At the same time, feel yourself in the space that surrounds your body, the energy of your life meeting the energy that's in the space near you and beyond. Enjoy the experience of feeling spacious and feeling yourself in space.

Slowly open your eyes. Continue experiencing feeling spacious and feeling yourself in space. Enjoy living in the space of your body and in the space around you as you go about the rest of your day.

Record and repeat

Repeat the Conscious Body Awareness exercise often during the course of reading this book. Notice the differences in what you experience each time. You can do the exercise to help you fall asleep or to help you feel grounded and energized. If you do this exercise in a group, discuss what you notice during the experience and how you feel after completing it. You can also journal about it.

To keep from having to repeatedly glance at the book each time, you can record the exercise instructions on a CD or tape and play them back to guide you through the process, or you can purchase my "Appreciate Your Body" CD with its recorded set of instruction for this exercise.

What Does Your Body Have to Say?

OBSERVE AND REFLECT

CONSCIOUS KINDNESS: Reflect on your experience of the Conscious Body Awareness exercise. Note one area of your body that caught your attention in particular, either because you weren't aware of much feeling in that area or because the feeling there surprised you or otherwise interested you. Promise yourself to treat this area with extra attention and kindness in the coming days. Then keep your word.

ENJOY YOUR HANDS: Spend time enjoying your hands (or choose another body part to enjoy). Quiet your mind for a few minutes, relaxing as much as possible using your favorite relaxation technique. Let your eyes soften. Gaze at your hands for at least a full minute. Look at them as if for the first time, as a baby might, noticing their shape, size, color, spots, lines, hills and valleys, movement. Consider the miracle of your hands and how they have affected your life. Who have they touched and held? What have they lifted, pushed, pulled? What has prompted them to applaud? What have they created? Who have they waved good-bye to? What injuries have they sustained? Remember the story of your hands. Thank them for all they have given you.

WRITE

WRITE WHAT YOUR HANDS LOVE: Write for five minutes, beginning with "One thing my hands love is . . ." or "Without my hands, I would miss . . ." If you're part of a group reading this book together, have each person read her writing aloud. Ask each person to contribute a line from her writing to create a group poem titled "My Hands." If you'd like, you can print out the poem and share it with friends and family.

BEGIN A MEMOIR: Let your writing be the beginning of a memoir or a legacy book you create for your family.

LIVE

DO WHAT YOUR HANDS LOVE TO DO: Think of something your hands used to love doing and find a way to do it again, if only in pantomime. Notice the pleasure this gives you, and let that feeling seep into your whole body.

HAND DANCE: Let your hands move freely to music you like. Create this "hand dance" by yourself or with a group. Enjoy the feeling of freedom and the beauty of the movements. If you're in a group, let everyone's hand movements join in a dance together. You can also let your dance expand into your whole body if you want.

HAND STORYTELLING: Develop a set of hand movements based on a story from your life and create a performance for children or other audiences, perhaps including puppets or other objects. Tell the story by letting your hands do much of the talking. The story could include lessons learned, or it could teach others in a fun way something of importance from your experience. Invite the audience to join you in some of the movements.

HAND MINDFULNESS: Spend a whole day being mindful of your hands. Observe them as you reach for a cup, wash dishes, pick up the phone, put a key in the door. Slow the motion down so each activity is done consciously, as a holy act. Thank your hands at the end of the day for their service and for giving you pleasure.

TAKE UP SPACE: Watch for instances during the week when people seem to "get in your space." Quiet your thoughts for a moment, breathe deeply, and bring your attention to the space inside your body and to the weight and full size of your body as it takes up space. By centering yourself consciously in the spaciousness of your own body, you may feel less need to act defensively. You'll have a sense of your own being giving you all the room you need.

CHAPTER 2

Knowing Your Body
as an Intimate Friend

Is your body too fat/ugly/short/wrinkled? Most of us can readily come up with a list of things we consider "wrong" with our body. That's how we were brought up—to be body critics. In our youth, the perfect size, shape, and complexion stared at us from the covers of *Seventeen* and *Glamour* and in all the ads, promising—no, demanding—to show up in our mirror. They never did, of course, and we learned from early on to give ourselves a critical eye in the mirror: *Oh, look at that flab on my arm—ugh! My breasts are the wrong size. Geez, I look funny.*

Even though we're well beyond our self-conscious teen years, the advertising industry makes sure the message stays with us: we *should* have a perfect body, but we don't. Now they woo us with skin creams and surgery to eliminate "unwanted" wrinkles and entice us with the promise of perfect abs to replace "unsightly" flab. Not that we need to be reminded of our body's supposed shortcomings. Our self-critic training from our early years has left a deep track on our psyches.

Anna, a petite dancer in her sixties who once performed professionally, now teaches dance and exercise classes. A woman in tune with her body, she easily outpaced and outgraced me when I accompanied her on her daily walk through her neighborhood. Yet she told me that the self-loathing anorexia that ran her life in her younger dancing years still calls to her, trying to reduce her down to the "right" size. Our body remembers the stories it has heard about itself from way back when.

Stop a moment and consider: Do you think there's something "wrong" with the way you look? How old is that opinion? Where did it come from?

It's not only our external appearance that we criticize. We blame ourselves for not being in top health. Once again, the ad industry makes sure we see ourselves as negligent caretakers of our body. We must not be taking enough of the right supplements, using the right medication, getting the right exercise, or sleeping in the right bed. The long and oft-repeated litany of what we're not doing right reinforces the "I've got it all wrong" song we began learning in our toddler years. Add to that the unsolicited advice of people who relish pointing out that our religious waywardness or emotional dysfunctions are "causing" our health problems, and we can quickly feel ourselves at odds with our body.

We're disconnected from our body

Feeling somatically disconnected comes easily to us anyway. Most of us didn't learn how to love living in our body when we were growing up. Instead, we were taught the importance of the mind—for acquiring facts, for analyzing and categorizing, for judging and making choices. The well-schooled mind was to dominate the body, which was let out to play less and less often as we got older. In school, we learned to keep still and quiet—moving and speaking only when told to do so or when playing organized sports. For the most part, we left our body and lived in our mind. In social settings, our body was to be decorated, entertaining, and alluring. At the same time, religion told us to subdue our body to reach enlightenment or for the salvation of our soul. Some of us suffered from harsh parenting or other forms of abuse that left us with averting eyes, drawn-in chests, and "I'm sorry" as our mantra.

In the midst of all these constraints, our body developed protective strategies for survival—patterns we may still carry with us. In our teenage and later years, some of us sought ways to break free from these restraints and unleash somatic feelings of freedom and pleasure. A good many of us turned to alcohol, drugs, sex, or excessive eating (or starving) to do so. As we got older, many of us eventually succumbed to busyness—the mercilessly demanding god in our restless society that presses us to be constantly in action. If an urge or a pain in our body asks for our attention, we may pop a pill or down caffeine and keep on moving instead of listening to what our body is asking of us.

We hunger to feel at home in our body, to enjoy living in it, yet we may look outside of ourselves to fill ourselves and soothe our hurts. Maybe our body is crying out for attention rather than action. We may already be *full* but just haven't spent time exploring what our core, authentic fullness feels like.

All of these approaches that subdue, dull, or artificially pump up our body ultimately distance us from it. These approaches keep us from paying attention to our body's real needs and wants. By midlife, however, our body begins to demand our attention. Menopausal upheavals, "bad knees," vision losses, and other bodily pains and challenges confront us. And the response once again often comes from the inner critic. Too often I've heard women say, "This damn body—it doesn't do what I want it to do" or "I hate my body."

Part of the reason we're ill-equipped to respond to the cries of our body is that we are somatic illiterates. Even after living in our body for all these years, we hardly know it. We've learned to regard it as a servant rather than as an intimate. We expect our body to do our mind's bidding and to hold up well regardless of how we treat it. We rarely stop to get acquainted with our body to find out what it knows or desires.

Don't wait until you're dying

How would you like to make friends with your body? What might it feel like to turn off the inner critic and treat your body with respect, with unconditional love?

In her book *The 85th Year,* Edith Mucke, near the end of her life, reflects on what it has meant to live in her body for a whole lifetime, calling her body "my house." She writes, "I was born in this house, built in the womb of my mother. I will die in this house." Her body, she writes, "has many rooms all safe and connected, held together by a complex structure of bones, sinew, muscles, joints, empty spaces (lots of air), and lots of water."

We do not need to wait until we are dying to make ourselves at home in our body. We can start now.

Develop curiosity and gratitude

In chapter 1, you learned some ways to get better acquainted with your body by sensing what it feels like to live—to be *alive*—inside your body. By cultivating childlike curiosity, awe, and gratitude, you can further strengthen your friendship with your body.

Your physical form is beautifully designed and remarkably complex. Billions of cells perform billions of operations every day on your behalf. Right this second, countless messages are leaping between the synapses of your brain, giving minutely detailed guidance to every area of your body. Your respiratory and cardiovascular system are collaborating in an intricate set of interchanges to supply your body with just the right amount of oxygen while disposing of carbon dioxide and other wastes. An array of hormones are circulating through your blood, each of them smart enough to know which specific cells need them. As they attach themselves to these cells, proteins are synthesized, enzymes are activated, or a host of other changes alter their workings. What marvels your body performs to keep you well and active!

Awareness of such wonders can't help but inspire awe. But how can this sense of awe become routine? Again, wide-eyed curiosity and appreciation are good starting points.

Thrill to the miracle of hearing

One day I met a woman at the beginning of a class we were both taking. "I'm Jeannie and I'm deaf," she announced with a big grin that exhibited both kindness and a sure sense of herself. (She obviously wanted to help me feel at ease communicating with her.) Her vibrant self-respect and generosity spurred me to reply with laughter, "Good to meet you. I'm Pat and I can hear." She laughed with me, recognizing that she had prompted me to remember what a joy it is to be able to hear. I felt exhilaration for the next few days over the many sounds I took in.

I remember a similar experience of delight in the gift of hearing. After a luxurious hike with a friend near the shore of Lake Superior in northern

Minnesota, I plunked myself down on rocks right next to the tumbling waters of Gooseberry Falls. The whooshing rush of water is one of the sweetest sounds on earth. As I listened, rough spots got washed over and worn away. My body and soul felt refreshed, sated. I walked away lighter, unrushed, serene.

How grateful I was that day for my ability to hear. While I sat there, still and unmoving (I thought), this ecstasy was being created by thousands of tiny hairs deep inside my ears. They picked up the water's sound waves and vibrated, dancing and singing the song of the water so I could experience it.

What a miracle that I can hear, I thought! Even more amazing is that my body carries a lifetime of recordings such as this waterfall symphony, which I can recall at will. A little prompt—such as turning on a faucet, seeing a smooth rock, or even imagining myself sitting again on those rocks—can get those hairs doing their dance and bring me to a state of contentment. How many wonderful memories we have, brought to us by our ears, that we can draw on to create a pleasant day.

What pleasure have your ears brought you today? If you're deaf, what other sensations can you pay close attention to?

Slow down to appreciate

We don't always appreciate something we have until we lose it. We tend to take the abilities of our body for granted. After I recovered from a bout with Lyme disease a few years ago, I felt rushes of gratitude as I reclaimed everyday abilities. I delighted in the first moment I could again lift my head without discomfort, walk across the room with full strength, cook my own meals, and dance. Years earlier, after a hand injury healed, I had a similar experience. I remember being thrilled at the ability to clap again while attending a concert. Sometimes the gift of illness is to unleash appreciation—to meet our body and our life with new awe.

Conscious attentiveness to our miraculous body rarely takes place when we're in a hurry. It's a meditative practice, most effective when done in a state of stillness. That doesn't mean we have to go off to a monastery or spend hours in the lotus position to learn appreciation for our body and sensitivity to its needs. I found the gift of stillness in the midst of illness and injury, which allowed me the opportunity be more conscious of my body's gifts. In general, we tend to be more alert to the needs of our body and its overall state of being when our health is weakened.

Look for the wonder of health

There's no need to wait for illness, however, to gain this state of attentive stillness. Look for opportunities to increase your awareness in your day-to-day activities, especially at times when you're already tending to your body's care. During a breast self-exam, for example, go beyond checking for signs of cancer and look for signs of health. Thank your breasts for the joy and pleasure they have brought you and for the ability they have given you to nurture children.

What about appreciating your joints while you prepare for your day? Thanks to the cooperation of your joints, you can bend over and pick up your morning newspaper, shower and wash your hair, dress yourself, make yourself breakfast, and sit down and eat it. Imagine how different life would be if your body were one solid mass, without the ability to bend!

Make good use of visits to the doctor for those uncomfortable "preventive" procedures. Your attention is already directed toward your body—so what a perfect opportunity to get better acquainted with some of its less well-known parts.

One of the most feared (and avoided) health checkups is a colonoscopy. I rarely give much thought to my colon unless it isn't working well. I take for granted that it will "eliminate the negative," and I don't much like the smell coming out of it. That's usually about as much attention as it gets from me. But when I had my last colonoscopy, I got a splendid view of the inside of my colon on the monitor next to me. As the doctor finished his work and his scope rapidly retreated through my colon, it looked to me as if the colon's thick pink soft-sculpted walls were doing the moving, rolling by in wavelike motion as fluidly as seaweed under water. I was truly surprised by how beautiful they were.

In preparation for my colonoscopy, I had to empty it out completely. "Empty yourself," the Buddhists say. Okay, I decided, I'd make this a spiritual exercise while I was at it. I was fearful about going without my usual foods. I didn't like the prospect of getting hungry and weak, of feeling "empty." I became aware again, as I have often done over the years, of how much I turn to food for more than physical nourishment. Some people can forget to eat or easily go most of the day without eating. Not me. I tend to think about food a lot—too much—and I tend to overindulge. One more bite turns into one more bowl. When the meal is over, my thoughts go to, "What else can I eat?" I eat healthy foods, mind you, but I've learned that even healthy foods don't turn off a food-addicted brain like mine. Much like booze for an alcoholic, food can easily take control of my life. My eating compulsion requires daily surrender to a Higher Power if I don't want my day to be ruined by binging.

So, emptying out my colon is no small thing. Neither is fasting. That "emptiness" makes me more vulnerable—physically, emotionally, and spiritually. In preparation for my colonoscopy, I chose to welcome that vulnerability and find out what gifts it had to offer. I know that emptiness can actually be "filling," because it sharpens my senses and raises my alertness. My way of seeing and acting becomes clearer. Once I couldn't eat, I particularly noticed that I smelled food more keenly. And since I couldn't eat what I smelled, my attention turned to the pleasantness of the aroma. I enjoyed the fragrance for its own sake, rather than focusing on getting the food for myself. There was peace in that rather than compulsion.

That same pure sense of enjoyment came through as well when I saw my colon walls. Another day the sight may have struck me as ugly, but under the influence of emptiness, the beauty of this body part that is seldom seen or discussed appeared beautiful.

Appreciation improves your health

Appreciation for our body is not just a "nice" thing to do. Such appreciation actually changes our body. Science has shown us that even the simple act of observing something changes its molecular structure. So does directing thoughts or words toward it. Japanese researcher Masaru Emoto has illustrated through dramatic photographs that words and thoughts change the molecular makeup of water. Water that is prayed over forms a well-defined, spectacularly beautiful crystalline structure. When words of love and appreciation are spoken near the water, the effects are similar. By contrast, negative words spoken near the water dissipate the crystals or generate amorphous clusters. Since the body is made up mostly of water, a logical leap is to assume that its makeup is also affected by our thoughts and words. Research is underway to learn more about such effects.

Scientists at the Institute of HeartMath, in Boulder Creek, California, have shown that positive feelings improve our health. When we're under stress, directing attention to our heart and then recalling sincere feelings of love and appreciation shifts our physiology. Doing so helps to balance our heart rhythms and nervous system, and creates more coherence between the heart, brain, and the rest of the body. HeartMath has developed a five-step process for doing this effectively, called Freeze-Frame®, which includes asking your heart for a more efficient perspective on the stressful situation. Doing the Freeze-Frame technique repeatedly builds up an accumulation of calm, balance, and clarity. You can learn how to do Freeze-Frame from the book *The HeartMath Solution* by Doc Childre and Howard Martin and from other HeartMath resources. HeartMath's research has shown that this technique reduces cortisol (a stress hormone) levels and increases levels of the anti-aging hormone DHEA, among other healthful effects. The research results from HeartMath studies are awe-inspiring. They reiterate the power of appreciation.

What can happen if we direct our appreciation to the body itself? Myrtle Fillmore, the co-founder of the Unity movement, offers us an excellent role model. She describes in her writing how she cured herself of tuberculosis by spending extended periods of time each day blessing specific parts of her body and thanking them for their wonderful work. She speaks in *Myrtle Fillmore's Healing Letters* of claiming her birthright as a child of God. Because of this relationship with God, she came to the conclusion that her body did not inherit sickness, and she saw her body not as sick but as the perfect expression of God's life in her. She said she continued "blessing my body temple until it manifested the innate health of Spirit."

In January 2006, I lay in a hospital bed for the third time in less than a month, having survived a simple heart procedure but having endured many complications, including a zany prescription-drug side effect that left me "tripping" and then crashing. The timing of this medical disaster was particularly bad. I was in the midst of the launching of my book *Body*

Odyssey and intended to be completely immersed in its promotion. But there I lay, unable to speak or eat or move around because of the medical complications. I was crazed from the medication and panicking about how I would pay the sizeable portion of my medical bills not covered by insurance. And what about the long list of upcoming talks and workshops on my calendar? Would I have to cancel them all and suffer more income loss? In the middle of the night, I was restless and couldn't get to sleep. I felt a profound sense of despair and loneliness.

It was then that I remembered Myrtle Fillmore's body blessings. I also thought of all I had written and spoken about publicly regarding tapping into body wisdom. It was time to walk my talk. One of my beliefs is that whatever we pay attention to increases. So I decided to quit paying attention to all the negative thoughts swirling through my mind. Instead, like Myrtle Fillmore, I started to bless and appreciate my body. My way of doing this was similar to the Conscious Body Awareness exercise in chapter 1, but this time my thoughts were more active. Scanning my body very slowly, beginning with my feet, I contemplated and marveled at the gift that each part of it offers me. My thoughts went something like this:

....

How splendid that I have feet. What a miracle the way they are formed, with all their bones and muscles and tissues. How flexible my feet are. They hold me up, help me stay balanced, and move me where I want to go. They make it possible for me to walk, kick balls, dance, and step on car and bike pedals. They have allowed me to hike up mountains in Glacier National Park, walk through the Palmer Lake Preserve in my own neighborhood, move through stores with ease so I can get my groceries, climb up the long flights of stairs on Yucatan pyramids, run to catch a plane. Thank you, wonderful feet, for all the places you take me, all the fun you make possible, all the chances you give me to be with people I want to spend time with. I'm glad you support me so beautifully. I love and appreciate you, my feet.

....

Each part of my body—knees, hips, genitals, spleen, kidneys—received similar loving attention for several minutes apiece. It wasn't long before my troubles completely disappeared from my awareness. I had become attuned to the many activities going on in my body and to the many ways my body helps me enjoy life and express myself. As the appreciation grew within me, so did my sense of well-being. My body felt light and refreshed, opening me to what I can only describe as an experience of the Divine. An overwhelming feeling of peace settled over me. I was flooded with memories of God at work in my life, generating quite surprising and satisfying solutions in troubling times. From these recollections emerged a sense of ease about my future. A grin of anticipation spread across my face as I looked forward to the new ideas and help that I was now sure awaited me in the days ahead. I thanked God for my body and for what was to come, and then I easily fell asleep.

What Does Your Body Have to Say?

OBSERVE AND REFLECT

BODY APPRECIATION: Starting with your feet, spend time reflecting on and appreciating each part of your body. Remember the many positive experiences you've had with each area. Savor the memories. Feel the emotions from those experiences again. Picture the scenes. Recall the sounds, the movements, the sensations of touching or tasting. Express your appreciation for each area of your body. For those areas where you are less aware of the experiences (such as the spleen, perhaps), use your imagination to see or feel that area of your body in action as much as you're able. Don't strain though. Make this an experience of delighting in your body and feeling your gratitude and care for it. Create a CD of this meditative exercise for yourself, or make use of the guided exercise on my CD "Appreciate Your Body."

A TRIP INSIDE YOUR BODY: Close your eyes and take an imaginary trip inside your body. Begin at your vulva. Picture yourself as a miniature explorer or photographer with a flashlight and camera entering into your vagina and moving up through your internal organs, much as you would explore the tunnels of a cave. As you move through them, explore their color, shape, size, texture, temperature, and movement. Be curious. Let your imagination and sense of pleasure take over. Keep exploring as long as you enjoy doing so.

CHANGE YOUR MIND ABOUT YOUR BODY: In a group, discuss the ways each of you have considered your body "wrong" and how you came to that opinion. One by one, declare a change of opinion. Dance together to share your newfound appreciation for, and enjoyment of, your body.

WRITE

APPRECIATION LIST: Any time you're feeling blue or having health challenges, make a long list of what you appreciate about your body. Take one of the items on your appreciation list and elaborate on the wonders of this aspect of your body.

WRITE A SONG: Comedian Allan Sherman often wrote songs about body parts. One I'm reminded of says, "Your spine looks divine, exactly like mine." Write a song or a poem—serious or funny—about your divine spine. This can be an inspiring and fun exercise for a group to share.

THANK-YOU LETTER: Write a thank-you letter to your tongue, fingernails, knuckles, tendons, or some other specific part of your body.

APOLOGY LETTER: Write a letter of apology to your body or to any part of your body that you've thought of or treated as "bad" or "wrong" over the years, just as you would do to a friend whom you have mistreated. Avoid condemning yourself in the process. Instead, acknowledge that you didn't fully understand what a treasure your body is and that you now know better.

CELEBRATE RECOVERED HEALTH: Remember a time when you were ill or lost a physical ability and then recovered. Write about the experience of being able to resume normal activity again.

CREATE A BODY CREDO: In a group, have each person write and share a credo celebrating her body's wonder and beauty.

LIVE IT

MIRROR APPRECIATION: When you glance in the mirror at the start of your day, greet your body as your friend. Remind your body how beautiful, perfect, and precious it is. Make a promise to appreciate and take excellent care of it all day long.

MINDFUL EATING: Notice when you reach mindlessly for food or beverages. Wake up! Shift into conscious awareness and take in (or don't take in) the food or beverage in a way that honors your body's true needs.

IMAGINE YOURSELF WELL: When you feel a bodily discomfort or experience illness, hold an image in your mind of your body being completely healthy and easily able to do all the things it is meant to do. Return to that image again and again. Ask your friends to join in that prayer (your thought is a form of prayer), or do this in a group. If it fits with your religious beliefs, also remember your perfection as a child of a loving Creator. As you continue this practice over days and weeks, observe any changes in your well-being.

MOMENTS OF STILLNESS: Create moments of stillness and emptiness often during the day. In this state of being, scan your body and find an area to get to know better and appreciate. Enjoy, celebrate, and bless that area. Make plans to give it what it needs. This is a great exercise to do while waiting at stoplights or in a checkout line or when filling your gas tank. If you want to experiment even further, consider the notion that stillness and emptiness are our primary state of being—our essence—and that all our activity emerges from this state. Explore how your body feels and acts during the day when everything it does begins with stillness and emptiness.

CHAPTER 3

Whose Body Are You Living In?

Have you ever looked in the mirror and seen the face of your mother or father? Do you have the same vocal inflections as one of your parents, your siblings, or others who raised you? When I laugh loudly, I hear my sister's laughter ringing through my vocal cords. Who do people say you sound like or look like?

Your body has an ancestral history

Chances are that your voice, your way of walking, and many of your other bodily features resemble those of your parents, grandparents, and perhaps ancestors several generations back. Some of the resemblance is genetic. Facial features, skin color, and other DNA-based qualities are built in. My big ears came from my father's side of the family. What is your family's hand-me-down biology? Your DNA also includes genetic predispositions to certain health conditions, ranging from alcoholism to Alzheimer's. You carry your ancestral history in your body. This is true even if you've had little or no contact with your biological relatives since infancy, though you may not know the specifics of this inheritance.

What did your mother always say?

Beyond your DNA, you have certain qualities in your body that developed because of what you heard over and over again as a child. Your parents' repeated insistence that you "Sit up straight" and "Don't slouch" may have contributed to you having a beautifully erect carriage or a rigid torso, depending on their attitude and tone of voice when giving the instructions. Familial lectures that advised you to "Speak up and let people know what you think" may be one reason you have a healthy assertive manner. Or that message may have instead led you to feel shame about your shyness and avert your eyes every time you state your opinion.

What admonitions or words of encouragement did you hear again and again as a child? Were there unspoken guidelines? What did your mother or father always say? How have they shaped the way you move, hold your body, or speak?

Isn't it cute when she tilts her head like Grandma?

Some of your body's characteristics resulted from copying what you saw and heard around you as a child. Kids are great mimics. If your mom and your older sisters walked around with their chests stuck out in a "Don't mess with me" posture, you may have imitated them often enough to adopt the same stance as your own. Or maybe you mimicked this family attitude by acquiring extra weight in order to take up more space and keep people at a distance. You may still roll your eyes, sigh, talk fast, or put your hands on your hips just like one or both of your parents did.

What are the physical postures and expressions that you've adopted from your family members or others who raised you? Some you may like. Some may embarrass you. Some may make you laugh. I've chuckled numerous times when I've recognized my family quirks in myself. Yet at the same time, I'm very reluctant to admit that I'm "just like" someone else in the family.

My family mumbled. Well, not my mother especially; her volume became noticeably unimpaired when I didn't "get in here right now!" Nor my father, whom I remember as silent for the most part (maybe he did mumble and I just never knew it.) But my brothers (who outnumbered Mom and Dad by three)—there's no question that they mumbled. I remember my mother's exasperation when she couldn't hear them: "I don't know why you kids can't speak up."

She was right. It was hard to hear their mutterings, which were heard seldom enough as it was. Only one of my older brothers said much at all, and always in a mumble. He still mumbles to some degree. Whenever I talk with him by phone, at least once or twice during the conversation I find myself pressing my ear hard against the phone and covering the other one, straining to hear. It reminds me of the kind of bad connection we often had on long-distance calls when I was a kid, the kind during which most every call began with, "Can you hear me? Can you hear me?" But this fuzzy connection has nothing to do with phone-service limitations; the problem is my brother's mumbling.

I'll say, "So, what's new with you?" And I'll hear, "Nothing much. We got a half-inch of rain yesterday, so I couldn't . . ." My ear-pressing-to-the-phone starts. It's like his voice got lost inside his mouth somewhere and can't find its way out.

Now, I don't mumble. At least, I never thought I did until recently. I just speak softly. People tell me my voice is calm, soothing. Well, all right, maybe it is that, too. It is a quiet voice, for the most part. Too quiet, at least, for some voice-mail systems. You know the kind, the ones that are voice-activated and cut you off when they no longer pick up a sound. Well, I keep getting cut off after just a few words. I'm not loud enough to be heard.

That's not the first feedback I've gotten that I'm hard to hear. Several friends have told me they have trouble hearing me, especially on the phone, and I certainly can't blame that on a poor phone connection. On a recent call, I asked an artist friend if he had a taste for seeing an upcoming art exhibit with me, and he replied, "You're hungry for artichokes?"

Evidently I do mumble.

How did our families get to be this way?

How did our kin come to speak, walk, and talk in the manner they passed down to us? Beyond genetics, they were shaped by what happened to them and the meaning they made from those experiences. Collectively, the conclusions they drew from their experiences formed a family mythology—a set of beliefs and attitudes about themselves, the world, and the way life works. A family's ethnic background helps to shape this mythology. People of Swedish origin, for example, typically express little emotion, based on the belief that being emotional is a sign of weakness. Strength and endurance are highly valued in Swedish culture. This way of looking at emotions probably goes back many generations. Who knows exactly its origins, but it affects the people born into that culture, shaping their behavior and even their bodies. The quiet, reserved manner of speaking and moving are hallmarks of Swedes and other Scandinavians, exemplified in the stories of radio host and author Garrison Keillor's Lake Wobegon.

Ethnic culture is only one of many influences on a family's mythology. Religious beliefs, income level, geographical region, health, occupation, family tragedies, and other factors contribute to every family's outlook and its physical expressions.

We often adopt not only the physical expressions of our family but also the thinking or mythology behind them. John, a guy with bulky, rounded shoulders, was experiencing a great deal of back pain. In a workshop I co-led, John participated in an exercise in which, with eyes closed, he took backward steps, imagining himself stepping back into the bodies and mindsets of his father, grandfather, and great-grandfather. John came from a family of miners, and as he "entered" their bodies, he felt the effects of their backbreaking work. He later told me, "The men before me were used to bending down to go into the mine. That must be how they felt about life. You had to bend down and go to work, and there was no way out. And that's the way I've been feeling in my life, like it's all hard work, like it's this huge burden. No wonder I have back problems. I remember my dad and my uncle walking around bent over. And now I'm doing the same thing."

John's body bore witness to his family legacy. Once he was aware of what the men in his family had believed and embodied, he could appreciate more fully how it had literally shaped him. He could also begin to reshape his outlook in ways that could lift the "burden off his back" and thus reshape his body as well.

In a Body Odyssey class I taught, a group of African American women in their sixties and seventies stepped back into the experience of their female ancestors, using this same guided process. They "remembered" in their bodies the long days of labor in the fields, the demeaning treatment of the slave masters, the responsibility of raising large families. After doing this exercise, these women were eager to tell stories of their mothers and grandmothers and how their ancestors' experiences had shaped their own lives. One woman spoke of how excited she had been as a child to be able to help her mother in the cotton fields—and how hard she had worked. She recounted an incident when she had picked so much cotton in one day that the overseer didn't believe it was all hers and refused to pay for all her work. A brave elder stood up for her and insisted she be paid what she deserved.

After the storytelling, I put on music and the women began to dance. They let this newly embodied sense of their past be told through movement. I watched as their bending and sweeping movements told of working in the fields, chopping wood, carrying babies, and much more. Their stories of struggle were apparent, but so was their robust patience, determination, and communal caring. The dancing continued for a long time, emerging into a full-bodied celebration of past and present, misery and beauty, struggle and triumph. Like John, these women, too, found a new sense of themselves and their past by letting their bodies have their say.

In more ways than one, your body carries your ancestral history. It is filled with stories. How wonderful when we listen to our body!

Family beliefs and habits may affect your health

You may even share illnesses with your family. Genetics plays a role, but we also pick up family eating, smoking, drinking, and other habits that influence our health. Family beliefs and values leave a legacy as well. Depression runs in families. So does high blood pressure. And cancer. Attitudes and beliefs may contribute to these tendencies. We can never assume, of course, that a certain disposition or set of values is the cause for any particular person's illness. But I can't help but wonder if the perfectionism so prominent in my family has been a factor in the high rate of heart problems among my siblings and me. The emphasis on getting things right certainly pushed us to work overly hard, creating undue stress. With "hurry up" as our family's mantra, a tendency to rush took up residence as tension in my neck and back muscles, and more than the needed amount of adrenaline and cortisol is regularly cued up. No doubt this tendency overworks my heart when it tries to keep up with the frantic pace. This family tradition probably contributed not only to the heart problems but also to the back pain, TMJ, and other ailments common in our family.

What are some of the prominent beliefs and values in your family ancestry? How have they "shaped" your body? Your health?

You can feel them when they walk in the door

Along with all the influences on our body from family and other important people, we are also linked to these people energetically. If my dad walked into the house while I was practicing piano as a child, he said little if anything, but I quickly stopped playing. I knew he didn't like "all that racket." I *felt* and complied with his spoken and unspoken demand for quiet.

When I was married, I could feel my husband's mood permeating the house. I'm sure my mood did the same, but I was more aware of the influence of his mood on my well-being. When he was angry, his whole body exuded this emotion. Around this intense negative energy, I would get tense and I'd tire easily, whether or not we had any discussions related to his anger. By contrast, when he was in a good mood, I was more at ease.

A few years ago, I had a young man as a housemate, and we'd often comment on how much we were affected by each other's emotional state. If he was confused and distracted by something that was on his mind, even if he didn't talk about it until later, I'd have difficulty concentrating myself. When I was upset by some experience I'd had during the day, he'd feel the energy of my emotion in the house the minute he came in the door, even before he saw me. By the same token, I have several friends who have a very calming influence on me without their having to say a word.

Do you pick up the "vibes" of the significant people in your life? Perhaps at times you even register pain or excitement that isn't yours.

A middle-aged dentist told me about an incident that illustrates this point in an extreme way. She was at work one morning when she suddenly felt sharp pains in her left hand. By midday, her hand hurt so much that she could hardly move or use it. At the end of her shift, she learned that her son had been rushed to the hospital with a cut in his left hand from a knife. Her hand pain continued even after she saw her son, who by then had received treatment, including pain medication, and no longer felt any pain in his own hand.

Still in touch even after they're dead

Even after people die, their energy can sometimes influence us. Following a workshop I gave about the lessons of the body during grief, a short, dark-haired woman with a strained expression on her face came up to me. In a hushed tone, she asked me, "Have you ever heard anyone talk about strange things happening after someone dies?" I could tell she was clearly bothered by some experience she'd had and wanted to talk about it.

When I assured her I had indeed been aware of unusual experiences around the time of death, she told me a lengthy story about her mother's final illness, and of being awakened in the middle of the night a few days after her mother's death by a feeling of enormous pressure on her stomach and on other parts of her body—the same parts of the body where her mother had had tremendous pain prior to dying. The woman, frightened, had awakened her husband to report this experience to him and then, within a short time, told him about the pressure suddenly leaving and the tremendous sense of peace she felt flood through her. Was this normal, she wanted to know? She was sure she wasn't crazy. She *knew* this had happened.

Many women have reported similar experiences on my blog. One woman, while washing dishes, felt the warm, firm hug of her grandmother from behind her. The grandmother was miles away, dying. Another woman, long after her husband was dead, felt the reassuring presence of his body lying on hers—not in a sexual way, but as a comforting presence. Other people have told me about hearing a dead loved one's laughter or of experiencing the person's touch. Everyone's body appears capable of being an active channel for the energetic expressions of others, living or dead.

Meet the family

How much influence have your family and other people had on your body? The answer might be worth knowing in order to deepen your friendship with your body. Paying attention to this can be an important step in ridding yourself of those influences that are undesirable and in celebrating those who you cherish.

You need not be bound by your family history and mythology. No matter which messages you took in and embodied, if they don't contribute to your well-being now, you can change them.

EXERCISE: THE "HOWEVER CLAUSE"

One way to make this change is to use the "however clause." Let's say one or more of your ancestors experienced a painful betrayal. Maybe a spouse had an affair or a brother misused family money in secret. As a result, a core belief may have developed in the family that "you can't trust anybody." This belief may have permeated your family life while you were growing up, so much so that it has shaped your thinking and behavior without your even realizing it. You may have been taught to keep things a secret for fear that someone would take advantage of you, or you may have become constantly watchful of other people for signs that they're trying to "get one over" on you. Your body could give you clues about this ingrained way of thinking—a vigilant tension somewhere (or all over) or tightly closed lips (the origin of the term "tight-lipped," no doubt).

Once you recognize this core belief or mythology, you can add a however clause to it. Begin by stating (or writing), "I've always believed _____." (For example: "*You can't trust anybody.*") Now add a new perspective: "However, _____." (For example: "*That's not completely true*" or "*I don't believe that anymore. I now think . . .*")

The however clause is a simple way to begin moving from being the victim of your history and the resulting family mythology to being the creator of a new story that empowers and energizes you. The more you elaborate on your new way of thinking and the more you practice repeating it, the more likely you will experience its effects. If you have typically mistrusted people, for example, you may find yourself more willing to take people into your confidence or to get emotionally close to them, while still using reasonable caution when necessary.

Changing one's mythology usually involves more than using new words though. You have embodied the old myths for a long time. Paying mindful attention to your body's way of living out these myths opens the way to explore deeper and more lasting change. In later chapters, you'll learn more about how to let your body lead you into living the new story.

What Does Your Body Have to Say?

OBSERVE AND REFLECT

YOUR FAMILY INHERITANCE: The next time you are with members of your biological or adoptive family, observe their physical characteristics that are not exclusively related to their genetics:

- Posture—while standing, sitting, and moving about
- Vocal quality and volume
- Gestures
- Speed of activity
- Health problems
- Any other unique features

Observe which of these characteristics are reflected in your own body. Do this without judgment. If you have trouble noticing your own body habits, ask someone who knows you well to describe your non-genetic physical characteristics. If that person knows your family, he or she can help point out your similarities to your family members. If this is a person you easily can have fun with, ask him or her to demonstrate your features or behaviors, and have a good laugh about them together. If some of your characteristics bring up painful memories, you may want to explore them with a compassionate friend or a circle of women.

ACT OUT YOUR CHARACTER: Imagine you were going to play the role of yourself in a theatre play. How would you build this character? What beliefs and attitudes would she have? What physical characteristics would she exhibit? Make this a fun exercise. Act out a scene as this "character." Play it *big*. Exaggerate your behaviors. Don't try to change or "correct" anything. You're just exploring with curiosity the person known as you. If you're part of a supportive group you trust, have the group members offer you suggestions from their experience of you as you take on this role. Afterward, journal or discuss with your group how it felt to step more fully into your own "body" and the associated beliefs and attitudes.

WRITE

LIVE IN YOUR ANCESTOR'S SHOES: Choose one of your female ancestors (mother, grandmother, great-grandmother) and imagine living in her shoes for a day. Write the story of her day in the first person, from her perspective, describing what happens, what she thinks about it, and how she responds. As you write, try to live inside her body, feeling what she feels, moving as she moves. Imagine where she feels tension, energy, or pain in her body. When you are finished, write in your own voice about a recent day in your own life, again emphasizing your body's experience. How closely does your experience—especially your body's reaction—match your ancestor's?

WHAT YOUR MOTHER ALWAYS SAID: Make a list of phrases your mother always said that represent admonitions, advice, or a particular point of view. Do the same for your father's sayings. If you can't recall specific words they said, write key ideas or principles they communicated to you—the unspoken family myths. Notice how these messages live in your body. If any of those sayings or ideas don't match your current or desired beliefs, use the "however clause" to revise them so they do. Notice any differences in your body when you say these revised beliefs out loud.

LIVE

EXAGGERATE A FAMILY TRAIT: Occasionally exaggerate one of your family-learned characteristics for a whole day. The next day, exaggerate the opposite characteristic. Enjoy the range of behaviors this experiment gives you as you go about your daily life.

Part 2

Heal Your Body

"The journey to the bones, the organs, the interior, is one
a healer or sick person must take in order to seek a cure, as
if following illness back to its origins and remembering the
body history as a kind of map or story."

LINDA HOGAN, *The Woman Who Watches Over the World*

CHAPTER 4

Healing from Big Traumas

Most of us experience some form of trauma in our life—the sudden loss of a loved one, a car accident, the loss of an important job or a major dream, betrayal, a violent incident, a serious diagnosis. Many women endure intense and repeated abuse. These situations not only jar our psyche, but they also leave a mark on our nervous system and may produce other significant physical changes. If you've experienced trauma in your life, you may need professional help in order to heal these scars. You can also contribute to your healing by bringing compassionate attention to these scars and by honoring their stories in creative ways.

Trauma effects limit us

By the time I was in my early twenties, I had been in four car accidents. The first one happened when I was eight years old. A drunken driver rear-ended our family car as my mother slowed to make a turn, and our car rolled over several times into a ditch. That accident landed me in the hospital overnight. Not long after, I was riding with a family friend, and as we entered an intersection, a pickup coming toward us from the left failed to yield and smashed into the front section of my friend's car. While neither of these accidents resulted in major physical injury, I felt their effects for many years. Two accidents in my early twenties—one involving horses bolting out in front of our car at night and the other resulting from the failure of a car on a cross street to yield—intensified the trauma and left me too scared to get a driver's license until I was in my thirties.

I never would have thought of it as trauma during those years. I was not aware enough of my body to notice how deeply these experiences had affected me. I was briefly aware of feeling a "little shaken" at the time of these incidents, but they dropped out of my mind before long. They didn't drop out of my body, however. I can remember in my preteen and teen years the high anxiety that coursed through my nervous system and put my muscles on alert whenever a car in which I was riding approached an intersection. I'm not exaggerating: virtually every intersection I encountered appeared highly dangerous to me, and depending on the speed we were moving, my body went into varying levels of fight-or-flight preparation. I often took in a sudden sharp breath, making a *s-s-s-s* sound with my teeth. My feet would brace for a hit. I sometimes closed my eyes, threw up my hands in front of me, or gripped the side of the seat or whatever was on my lap. After a while, this pattern of gearing up for a possible accident became so common it felt normal, though the expression of my fear gradually subsided in its intensity.

At the time, I didn't recognize any of this as related to the accidents I had been in. In fact, as best as I can recall, I thought it was normal to feel the way I did. My body—from its stored memory of past danger—was communicating that intersections were dangerous, and my mind was influenced by this automatic assumption based on stored trauma, *even when the immediate situation showed no evidence that a car was likely to hit us.* It didn't help that my mother was also skittish about driving—perhaps in part because of her own experience of being hit from behind. I'm sure I picked up on some of her anxiety as well.

Your body registers the threats to your safety and security

How have you been "hit" in your life? If not in a car accident, perhaps you had a bad fall, were attacked or abused, or suffered some other physical or emotional blow. Maybe a significant love relationship ended. Perhaps you were fired or laid off, or your financial security evaporated. Maybe someone who mattered greatly to you died suddenly, spinning you into shock and immense grief.

Shocking and threatening experiences such as these jar our core sense of safety and security. The body, beautifully designed with an array of strategies to ensure our survival, gears up for self-protection. It generates a rush of chemicals and signals to alert us to danger and rally the necessary resources to ward off the threat. It sets up patterns of response—such as adrenaline rushing and muscles tensing for action—to help us keep safe and ready for action. When the threat is extreme or often repeated, these responses become like grooves in an old vinyl record. Our body interprets the threat as permanent or at least likely to reappear. Our internal system becomes organized to stay on continual alert or to gear up quickly at any sign of a renewed threat, whether that sign is real or imagined. The responses become automatic. Even when the threats are removed, the responses continue. Some of these responses may create ongoing tensions or chemical activities that eventually create pain, deplete or distort the body's resources, or lead to other dysfunctions.

What automatic, deeply grooved defensive responses remain in your body from your traumatic experiences? Where does your body feel on alert? What behaviors seem out of your control? What aches or illnesses are you experiencing that might reflect a self-protective stance?

Terror can make you forget you are loved

Scamp, my son's dog when he was a boy, was once picked up by the city pound after he left our yard. When he returned home, Scamp curled up in the corner of the yard and recoiled whenever I offered him food or called him to come play. Somebody had evidently treated him harshly while he was away, and now he couldn't trust even those who had always treated him well. It took almost a week of frequent, gentle reassurances and gradually moving closer to him each day before his frolicky, fun spirit was revived and we could all romp with him again.

Even though Scamp had been a much-loved dog, and he was back in the company of those who had cared for him for years, one instance of being traumatized nearly blotted out that whole history of good treatment, as far as his body was concerned. Fortunately, animals are quite resilient.

And so are we. But, as with Scamp, recovery from trauma usually takes a lot of nurturing attention and reassurances of safety, repeated over a long period, before trust can be restored and the body can return to normal or near-normal functioning.

Professional help restores safety and normalcy

If you have experienced severe trauma, you may need the help of a skilled therapist or other professional helpers to facilitate the process of recovery for you. Medications or nonmedical therapies may be necessary to reduce the effects of the trauma. Some traumas, such as extensive and repeated abuse or the experiences of war, may be so severe that, even after years of therapy and other interventions, remnants of the patterned responses can remain with you. In some cases, the trauma may have been so jarring that your mind shuts out some or all of the memory of what happened in an attempt to protect your psyche from the horrors of the experience. Yet the body remembers. Over time, signs of unhealed traumas such as frequent headaches, muscle tension, or night terrors may appear. Sometimes a hidden trauma can resurface quite suddenly, as happened in the case of my kidnapping.

When I was in my mid-forties, I attended a workshop designed to help people heal past hurts and find greater self-acceptance. At the beginning of the first session, as people were each taking a few minutes to introduce themselves and talk about the issues they wanted to address, I wasn't sure what I would say when it was my turn. I just knew I wanted to experience less anxiety in my life. However, much to my surprise, my body suddenly alerted me to an aspect of my anxiety that needed my attention. I describe this incident in the first chapter of *Body Odyssey:*

....

Bam! A noise explodes behind me. I jump a half-inch off of my cushion, my hands fly in the air, and my head whirls around to see the source of the disturbance. A folded metal chair has fallen to the floor. My whole body begins to shudder.

As my neighbor continues with her introduction, I try to stop my jittery moves, so as not to be distracting, to politely wait my turn, to avoid being noticed. But the trembling intensifies. Confusion, shame, fear, and heat envelop me.

After my neighbor finishes, there is silence. Cherie turns her soft eyes toward me. The whole group is watching. My eyes dart about; my gaze drops to the floor. I know my voice will tremble if I try to speak. I don't know what's happening to me or what to say.

Cherie speaks. "It looks like there might be something going on with you, Pat."

I try to make my jaw work. All I can do is shudder and nod.

"Would you like to talk about it?" She pauses. "You don't have to if you don't want to."

Somehow Cherie's permission not to speak allows me to do so, though my lips barely part: "I just got scared when that chair fell over," I say, as if that would explain my obvious terror.

"What was it about that chair falling that was so frightening?"

"I don't know. I can't figure out why it's bothering me so much. I can't stop shaking." The palsied tremors embarrass me.

"It's okay for you to be shaking here. We can try to find out what the shaking is about, if that's all right with you."

I nod, though I feel unsure.

"Did it remind you of something?"

···

Cherie wisely probed for clues. She was aware of how smart the human body is. It alerts us all the time to what needs our attention. Sometimes, such as when your stomach growls, the sign is simple and clear: your stomach's message is that you need to eat. But often, especially when emotional needs are involved, the clues require some Sherlockian sleuthing. This search for the "villain" requires patience and genuine curiosity. And sometimes metaphors, more than facts, reveal the path toward healing.

In the workshop incident, the sharp noise reminded me of a gunshot. Once Cherie asked the question, my memory quickly leapt to an episode five years earlier. One evening as I was getting out of my car in my garage, I experienced the horror of being abducted by a man with a gun. For almost two hours, I was held hostage until I was able to get him the money he wanted. Though the gun was never fired, a deep fear of being killed registered in my body as terror. I trembled intensely throughout the experience, and now, in this workshop setting, those tremors returned. I had more or less ignored those feelings in the days that followed the kidnapping, figuring they'd subside before long. They did subside, but my body continued to carry their memory in its cells. Five years later when I was prepared for healing work in the safe, compassionate setting of the workshop, my body reactivated the tremors as a way to signal me that I still had emotional scars from the kidnapping left to heal.

Those renewed tremors felt big and overwhelming. I didn't want to feel them, but there they were. I asked Cherie what to do with them.

....

"You don't have to do anything. Your body is already doing it. You just get to let the feeling be there, and I'll be right here with you to help you go through it. I'll help make it safe for you to have all the terror you've been holding in all these years, so you don't have to hold on to it anymore."

She invites me to lie down on the carpet and covers me with an afghan. I curl up in a semifetal position, shuddering and shivering all the while and trying to stop. Cherie places her hands tenderly on my shoulder.

"Now, Pat, just go ahead and let the fear be there, the big fear that your body is telling you about. You don't have to do anything but let your body do what it's doing. Your body is very smart and it knows exactly what to do."

For what seems like an hour, my entire body shakes and flails as if prodded by an erratic, low-level electrical current. There is no holding back. The shuddering and shivering take over. At times the movements become jerky, a vibration striking my legs or my shoulders like lightning. The shaking feels like it will never stop. From time to time, Cherie's assuring voice encourages me, coaches me.

"It's hard work to carry around so much terror inside. Let it come out now."

Cherie not only helped me release the long-standing terror and also bring up a waterfall of tears, she continued with the healing work by helping me find a strength within myself that could declare "no" to this kind of treatment:

"Your voice was shut down by having the gun pointing at you, but here there is no one to shut down your voice. So, Pat, you can say no here, you can tell this man who terrorized you to stop."

The tears and shaking subside a little as I consider her suggestion.

"No," I say weakly, wiping my eyes and nose of moisture. "No, don't do that." I feel foolish. He is not here now. But my body is shaking less.

"Why don't you sit up now so you can call up your full voice and say no." I feel ready to sit up and I do.

"See if you let your voice match the power of the terror and the grief and the anger you're feeling. Let it be louder. Let your 'no' be heard."

"No!" I am louder now.

"Good, Pat. Keep going. Louder."

"No! Stop that. Don't do that. Get away from me!" I'm not feeling foolish now.

"Good. Say, 'Get away from me' again, and let all the force of the terror you've been feeling back it up."

"Get away from me! Get away from me! Get . . . away . . . from . . . me! Stop it! Stop it! Stop it!"

"You have no right to do this," Cherie feeds me a line.

"You have no right to do this!" I am screaming now at the dark figure I remember. It is Larry, and it is not Larry. It is all the evil that moment came from and all that it created.

"I won't let you," Cherie offers another line.

"I won't let you. I . . . will . . . not . . . let . . . you. You will not do this to me. No! No! No! I hate it that you did this to me! I won't let you do it to me anymore! I won't let you."

My voice softens. I'm through yelling; now I've begun declaring with confidence. "I am free from you. I am free. You don't scare me."

I am now sitting fully upright on my knees. My voice is clear. I am not shaking anymore. I take a very deep breath. The room is quiet. My whole body is throbbing, not with terror but with a pulsing sense of power. I barely notice the enormous exhaustion and achy residue of unbridled terror and tears.

Cherie smiles tenderly. "That was very courageous, Pat—very beautiful."

Now I feel tears of relief welling up. "Beautiful." This seems like a strange word, but like milk from the breast, I drink it in.

"I wish you could see your face. It's radiant. It's beautiful."

How marvelous that there are therapists, teachers, bodyworkers, and other helpers who can guide us wisely and compassionately in listening to our body! As we find and express the deep truths within ourselves, our body emanates the natural beauty that Cherie alluded to. It exudes the radiance of authenticity. Our inner spirit shines through.

You may have had moments like this yourself, where a painful part of your past reappeared in some physical form, and with the help of a professional, you experienced a breakthrough leading to a sense of freedom and authenticity. Who did you find to help you bring that old experience to a point of completion and healing? What methods were used? If you are still experiencing some obvious signs of trauma, or if you're aware that you have some episodes from the past that still haunt you in a way you can't quite pinpoint, consider getting professional help. Many forms of assistance are available. Psychotherapy (especially body-based approaches), drama and dance therapy, Hakomi, and energy healing are just a few of the approaches that I've seen to be quite effective in cleaning house on the residuals of trauma. While it may seem frightening to consider revisiting the past and bringing up pain you'd rather forget, doing so in the presence of caring and competent professionals can give you the safety to move past those experiences to greater freedom and ease in your life.

Exercise: "Inner Champion" Writing

In addition to getting professional help, there is a great deal you can do yourself to unravel traumatic tangles from your past. Two activities that therapists often suggest, and that you can also do on our own, are journaling and "angry" letter writing. These activities can be enhanced by engaging your body's wisdom in the writing process. Let's say you plan to write a letter expressing your outrage to someone who treated you violently. This is not a letter you are actually going to send, but rather one that allows you to fully air your grievances without censorship. Later, you may read this letter to a therapist or another caring person who appreciates the pain of this experience and understands your need to give voice to your feelings about it.

One way to prepare for this writing exercise is to check in with your body. Find a place and time where you can be quiet and undisturbed. Become very still. You do not necessarily need to be totally relaxed, but do your best to bring your attention to the present moment and the experience of being in your body *now*. With the intention of writing your letter held in the background of your mind, slowly scan your body to locate some area that can represent the Champion in you—a part of your body that you can count on as a base from which you can take a stand. For example, maybe it's your feet as they rest firmly on the floor or your sturdy, dependable spine. Check to find your personal point of strength, wherever it might be.

This Champion does not have to feel like an aggressive fighter. It could have the feeling of a gentle giant or of a peaceful but strong advocate such as Gandhi. If this Champion doesn't feel very strong at the moment, take some time to recall—with full feeling—a past experience when its power was such that you felt invulnerable. It may be a time when you had a sense of certainty in your belly or a courageous, loving heart that felt like it could take on anything with ease. Soak in this memory as if bathing in it, feeling the physical and spiritual strength of this past experience as if it were present now. If you can't recall ever feeling strong in the past, think of a hero you've read about, seen in a movie, or known personally. Imagine what they feel in their body in moments of great courage and power, and bring up similar feelings within yourself. It helps to anchor these feelings in some part of your body.

Once you've connected as deeply as you can with this center of strength within yourself, ask this Champion to become your writing guide. You can either have your Champion do the writing for you, letting the words on the paper speak as if in your Champion's voice, or you can call on it for direction as you write in your normal way. As you express your feelings on paper, stay connected with the physical part of you that the Champion represents. Let the words carry the weight and power of this Champion strength. Write until everything you want to express is expressed. Then check with your Champion to see if there is anything more to say that would be for your good. Thank your Champion for being a source of strength and support during this exercise. Treat this part of your body with special appreciation in the hours and days that follow.

In the class I teach called Writing Your Own Permission Slip, I introduce activities like this one to help people draw on the wisdom of their bodies to revisit and revise the mythic stories they live by. In one session of the class, I invite participants to explore the "hero" in themselves—to physically remember those moments when they acted heroically in their lives. Some recall the type of heroism that makes headlines—saving a life or achieving an extraordinary athletic feat. But most reconnect with ordinary heroic acts—raising children, tending to a dying friend, going to graduate school, taking on a big volunteer project. Reliving such moments with a *felt* sense brings back into their minds and bodies the courage, resilience, determination, selflessness, and other heroic qualities they possessed at the time *and still have available to them.*

Because I came from a history of abuse, I always looked at myself as a survivor. After the class, instead of looking at myself as a survivor, I think of myself as a hero. It has really made a big self-concept change for me. I have lived with the identity I was given, and I couldn't seem to let it go because I was afraid then I would be nothing. But being a hero has a definiteness—a self to give myself instead of a nothing. A hero has real strength to help people. Now I feel the stuff I have to offer is coming out.

—Lola Wheeler, age 89

What are some of the heroic choices you have made in your life? How did you feel as you performed these acts? Where did that feeling reside in your body? Can you recapture that feeling now?

Throw the "damn you" eggs

Divorce is one of the most common traumatic experiences people face. Some people move through divorce with a certain amount of grace, but many people experience considerable shock, anger, and grief over the loss of this important love relationship. Complicating the loss may be financial upheaval or major conflicts about finances, the emotional disturbances of the couple's children, and a move to a new home. Collectively, these experiences can be traumatizing.

When I went through a divorce in my late forties, I gathered together a group of my closest women friends for a ceremony to help me bring closure to my marriage of twenty-one years. I invited them for a potluck meal at my home, and I also asked them each to bring along a dozen eggs—to throw. After these women arrived at my home, we went on a walk together to a nearby wooded area and used one of the trees as a target. I threw first. I wanted to make sure I got a chance to *physically* express the rage I had suppressed during my marriage. With each hurling motion, I let loose with an emotional blast: "If you won't help me, then just get out! Get out! I'm through with you." Then, the other women got their chance to vent frustrations in their own relationships. The sound of the "splat" on the tree was very satisfying for all of us, although we laughed more than we actually vented.

The silliness of it all almost dwarfed the seriousness of this attempt to unleash my pent-up tightness and terror. As a novice, I was clumsy at expressing difficult emotions. I wasn't used to standing up for myself—certainly not loudly. Yet I stepped forward as boldly as I dared, with friends as witnesses, and my whole body got into the act. As I had learned to do in Co-Dependents Anonymous, I was acting "as if," giving myself practice at the feeling of freedom.

It took another ten years and another egg-throwing outing with a friend before I allowed the full feeling of my rage to erupt. By this time I was more comfortable with my emotions and more at home in my body. When winding up for the tosses this time, a fire of fury surged up from my belly, and I was able to declare, "Damn you" and "Stop it! I won't let you do that anymore!" with the full force of my voice. As my emotional fury burst free of its confines, other emotions broke loose as well. Before long, my friend and I morphed our outbursts into a melody, and we were singing and laughing and staging a mini-musical, repeating, with increasing vigor, "Don't you tread on me!" as a refrain.

I have since heard of other anger-releasing rituals at the time of divorce. One woman told me that she and her friends drew life-size pictures of their former spouses, taped them to the side of one of the women's houses, and threw water balloons at them. As with the egg tossing, plenty of verbal venting accompanied the balloon hefting. What makes activities like this so effective is that the whole body gets involved. The emotional release comes up all the way from the bottom of the toes. There is also a certain kind of giddiness to it. The very silliness of the activity helps free up spontaneity and fun—uncensored freedom.

Give your story a stage

"People are usually surprised when I tell them that drama therapy can be fun and creative," Sheila Rubin, a Berkeley psychotherapist and drama therapist, told me. She leads ten-week sessions, called Life Stories Self-Re-velatory Performance workshops, consisting of body awareness and theatre exercises designed to help participants safely and creatively explore and heal emotional pain, including pain resulting from traumatic experiences.

In one of the exercises, participants gently massage and give attention to each area of their bodies, beginning with their feet. As they do this, Rubin guides them: "Ask your feet to remind you of the shoes you've worn. What kind of shoes were they? Where did your feet take you? Where have you walked, run, skied, or skated?" This gentle exploratory process helps participants become attentive to their bodies as reservoirs of memories. Rubin continues: "Ask your feet what stories they want you to remember." The participants in the group are learning to look to their bodies for sensations or for stories waiting to be told. After greeting, massaging, and learning from their bodies in this way, the participants talk about the stories they've reconnected with—maybe the memory of a grandparent teaching them to tie their shoes or a fun time playing football with a friend who has since died.

This story discovery process, based on body listening, is one of many exercises—some quite playful—that prepare participants for the final session of Rubin's class in which they do "self-revelatory performances," a form of drama therapy. At this session, each person tells his or her story in a dramatic form to invited guests. The person's history of struggle and longing, love and loss, and courage and triumph is given a stage. The story is told not only with words, but also with gestures, music, props, and other dramatic expressions that allow the performers to play out their experience as big as it feels to them. What helps to give meaning to this storytelling process is that the person is heard and seen by a community of supportive witnesses. Tears and laughter usually fill the room.

So often, this is what we hunger for—for someone to hear our story, to really *get* what we've gone through, and to understand what mountains we've climbed. Rubin puts it this way: "True healing requires a witness." Having others with "listening hearts" give us their full attention and honor our story validates our experience and assures us that we're not alone. Rubin emphasizes that, for victims of trauma, "coming out of isolation is really important." Giving our stories a dramatic staging is also creative and, as Rubin points out, "a creative act can be healing."

Perhaps your trauma feels so painful and personal that you can't quite bring yourself (yet) to expose your experience to a therapist, either alone or in a group of strangers. Or maybe you don't have therapy services nearby or the funds to make use of them. You may, however, be able to find self-help classes, workshops, and groups that offer opportunities for body-healing work and creative expression. Look for these listings in local newspapers, especially free health-and-wellness papers often available in urban and suburban locations. Ask for referrals from chiropractors, massage therapists, wellness coaches, and other professionals with knowledge of alternative healing approaches. Getting involved in improvisational theatre or dance activities or taking part in local theatre performances may allow you to explore your emotional sore spots. Look for play audition notices in your local newspaper want ads, or contact local theatres or dance companies to ask about the classes and workshops they offer.

Let a group support you

You can also create your own group, or find a friend who is willing to pursue emotional-healing activities with you. If you already belong to a support group, women's group, book group, or another group you trust, you may be able to do these activities with this group, or you can invite specific members to join you at another meeting time.

For years now, I have regularly met with one or more other people for weekly mutual support. My current group of three meets in my home, but other groups I've belonged to have met in each other's homes, at a church, or in a dance studio. The most important criteria I have when I look for a group, or form one myself, are criteria you might also wish to adopt. Consider seeking people who:

- Want to learn and grow emotionally and spiritually.

- Listen with heart, with full attention, and without judgment. In other words, find people who will hear you and love you as you grow. "Preaching," interrupting, and unsolicited advice-giving can quickly kill creativity in a group.

- Keep what is shared confidential. You can more readily share the secret parts of yourself if you know that no one will gossip about what you share.

- Make the group a priority. Regular attendance is important to keep everyone feeling connected and to understand each other's unfolding stories. If you've experienced trauma, it's especially important to have people you can count on.

- Are willing to engage their whole self in the group's learning and healing work. Talk alone is rarely enough to shift someone's core sense of herself. Attention to the body, including the use of creative expression activities, provides more entryways to healing and more ways to integrate it.

The activities you do in your group can be based on a book such as this one, a set of teachings you all agree to explore, or ones you create for yourselves. In my current group, we often start our meetings by spending a few minutes of silence to still our mind and connect deeply with the love and wisdom in our heart. We stir up feelings of love for ourselves or others and then ask our heart—yes, our physical heart—to guide us in what will serve the needs of our group for the evening. Because the heart is the physical center of our emotional life and because it emits an energetic frequency that has greater reach than even the brain, tuning in to what the heart knows and needs makes sense.

Also, the heart is often said to "break" or "close" after a trauma that has strong emotional elements. What better place to turn in order to learn what it will take to heal that break and reopen our heart. The heart is also a place where we can experience a sense of the divine at work. It may be the place where divine guidance can most clearly be perceived. In the group I meet with, whatever guidance each person receives during the time we tune in to our heart helps to shape the evening's agenda.

Focus on what your body is up to

One of the many types of activities our group has found helpful in these get-togethers is called Focusing. A process that gives us access to the body's knowing, Focusing was developed by philosopher and psychotherapist Eugene Gendlin. When we use Focusing in our group, one of us, with eyes closed, starts observing and describing aloud what she is experiencing within her body. She scans her body for sensations, impulses, aches and pains, temperature changes, emotional feelings, or anything else that is going on. She then focuses on the one thing that most strongly draws her attention, and follows it as it changes. It *does* change as she observes it, since attention to something always creates change.

As each of us is reporting her experience, the whole group serves as caring, attentive witnesses. We are *with* the participant, respecting her body's internal guidance, without any attempt to fix or suggest anything. One person in the group speaks back to her, echoing (paraphrasing) whatever she says, gently letting her know she is being heard and understood. If she says nothing for a while, the designated speaker for the group can ask, "What's happening now, ____(Mary)?" to prompt her to continue reporting. If she says, "I don't know," the listener can reiterate this experience with, "So, right now you don't quite know what is happening." Even the "not knowing" becomes an experience to observe.

This activity can take quite a while, and once the person senses that the group is with her and that there is no rush and no pressure on her for anything special to happen, she is free to follow with ease what is actually going on. Her curiosity becomes her guide. If she has had some kind of pain or tension going on for a while, it may intensify during this Focusing process. This is perfect. It's as if the painful area wants to have its full say. It wants to be heard, and now it's finally getting its chance, similar to the experience I had with the terror I was feeling in Cherie's workshop. Only when the trauma residing in the body is acknowledged in an accepting, caring environment can it begin to dissipate.

Sometimes images or thoughts come up for the person who is Focusing. They are often metaphors that give her insight into her discomfort. The image or thought of a bird trying to make its way out of an egg could be a clue that it's time for her to break free from something that has kept her small. If she keeps her attention on this image, it will likely change, and her feelings and sensations will change along with it. She may experience a mounting sense of "pushing through"—maybe in her shoulders or limbs—and eventually an expansive feeling of freedom.

Over and over, I have seen Focusing and similar body-attention processes lead people to significant relief from the effects of trauma. They experience much more than an intellectual "aha" moment. There is a change in the way they know themselves physically, emotionally, and spiritually. I have experienced this myself as a feeling of taking up more physical space and standing taller, along with having new levels of confidence and ease. The divine flows freely through me in those moments. I experience in body and spirit what it means to be one with God.

Bring yourself back to a state of trust

A woman told me that she'd had four car accidents in one year. Though they were not all her fault, she said she had lost trust in herself as a driver. I could easily relate to her due to the accidents I had been in, even though I wasn't the driver. Something in us gets deeply shaken when we are hit hard, whether physically or emotionally. We lose trust in ourselves and in the world (it's not operating in the way that it should). My car brakes once failed when the car I was driving hit a patch of ice I didn't see. I was confident the brakes would work—they always had. This time they didn't, and my car bumped the car in front of me. The panic I felt far outsized the accident.

Trust is a fragile thing. When you can't count on what you could always count on, there is a raw, naked, falling feeling—similar to when you lean against something that appears solid but isn't nailed down, and it gives way. You think you have planted yourself safely, but you haven't. I knew this feeling in a very pointed way behind the wheel of my car on the day my brakes failed. I pressed on the brakes and my sense of certainty gave way. I was greatly shaken by the experience. All the rest of that afternoon, a shrill, wailing cry was waiting to come out from a hollow, empty space inside me. Yet the cry remained unheard.

As the afternoon moved into evening, I stayed attentive to that falling feeling, the shakiness, and the unheard cry, all of which lingered. Something else about the failure of certainty seemed to be speaking to me through my body's fragile state, and I didn't want to miss its full meaning. I was spending the time at a party with old friends and my ex-husband—an awkward affair, and before long I recognized a parallel to my failed marriage, in which I had also felt as if there were "no brakes." I had trusted. I had expected the marriage to last, to remain solid. No matter how hard I had tried to hold off the dissolution of what I was once sure of, I could not. It was like being surprised by failed brakes. Trust would need to be rebuilt slowly, my wise body was reminding me that day. Once I got that message, I left for home and had a good cry. This new understanding didn't alleviate all my hurt and fear, but it did make a dent in my need to be "in control." It softened my fear of life's uncertainties. Healing from traumas often comes in small doses like that.

Trauma is something that happens to you that you don't expect, doesn't make sense, and wounds you deeply. Trust is eroded. But what you can count on, when it's over, is that your body knows the way out of this terror. If you give it your time and attention, eventually it will take you safely home.

Find a therapist, class, workshop, group, or friend to help you heal from your traumatic experiences. Use Focusing or other forms of body-based listening to identify and release whatever remains within you. Be kind to yourself and get the help you need. Don't delay. You deserve to enjoy your life without being weighed down by the burdens of the past.

What Does Your Body Have to Say?

OBSERVE AND REFLECT

TRAUMA CLUES: Make a list of circumstances or events in your life that may have caused you trauma. If you're not sure if a particular situation qualifies as "traumatic," add it to your list anyway. Review the items on the list one by one, and ask yourself for each item whether it's still a source of some stress for you. If you're not sure, notice any response in your body as you think about it. Do you feel tense or jittery? Does your chest sink, your jaw tighten, your brow furrow? Watch for the small signs of activity that may give you a clue about any effects of trauma that still reside in your body.

Whatever clues you discover, jot them down. Don't try to make sense of them for now, and don't judge them. Just take note of them for future use. For the next week, keep this list handy and continue checking in with your body throughout the day for further clues to jot down. Think of your-self as a detective, knowing that each clue is leading you to resolving a case that you will eventually close the book on. At the end of the week, thank your body for giving you these clues, and make a promise to yourself that you will explore what these clues have to tell you about your path to heal-ing. Then follow that path, using some of the activities described in this chapter (including getting professional help) or elsewhere in this book.

METAPHOR SEARCH: Make an appointment with yourself to tend to some persistent body discomfort, perhaps something you discovered in the exercise above. Observe the area of discomfort without trying to make it go away. Ask yourself what it reminds you of. Whatever comes to mind in response, ask yourself what *that* reminds you of. Keep going with this question until a memory or metaphor arises that greatly interests you. Consider what that memory or metaphor might be asking of you. What insight does it provide? What opportunity?

WRITE

INNER CHAMPION LETTER: Think of a person or group who contrib-uted to your experience of trauma. Write a letter expressing your feelings to this person or group. Seek a "Champion" within yourself to help you, as described earlier in this chapter. This Champion is most evident in some area of your body that carries your internal sense of strength and courage. To access the power of this Champion (which may be deeply buried), you may need to recall some past experience when the Champion actively gave you a sense of security and the freedom to speak up. Revisit that situation as vividly as you can in your mind and body, reactivating the thoughts, physical sensations, and emotional feelings associated with that experi-ence. If you can't recall ever having a Champion feeling, adopt one from a heroic person you've seen or read about. Make it your own. Write the letter in the voice of the Champion, or turn to your Champion as a coach while you write in your own voice. Share the Champion letter aloud with a person or group who will listen with heart and without giving advice. Pay attention to how your body feels after reading the letter.

LIVE

EGG TOSS: Get together with a friend or a group of friends and buy a supply of eggs. Find a place where you can safely throw them and where birds will clean up any residue. Make the outing as fun or as serious as you wish. Follow your instincts. Give your feelings full voice.

Chapter 5

Healing from Little Traumas

The stress you feel is not always the result of a major trauma. Your body also registers mini-traumas, or "little traumas," the occasional jolts or ongoing distress you feel from perceived threats. Maybe a parent, lover, or boss constantly demeans you. Or perhaps a bill collector is on your trail or you feel powerless to stop the health decline of someone you love. Whatever threatens your sense of safety or security can be traumatizing.

For more than twenty years, I lived in a part of town that I loved, but the crime rate there was the highest in the city. Right after I moved, I noticed how different my new neighborhood was. The streets were quiet at night—very quiet. No sounds of youths in the street or alley yelling and cursing. No breaking glass or screeching tires to wake me up with worries about possible crimes in progress. Rarely the sound of a siren. What I heard as I went off to sleep each night in my new setting was *nothing*. I remember how refreshing that felt the first night, and the second and the third.

In just a couple of weeks, I noticed a difference in my body, too. I felt an unfamiliar sense of relaxed ease. The constant vigilant tension that had kept me on alert for potential danger right outside my door, *a tension I had not been aware of*, was gone. I only noticed this long-standing tension because of its absence. When I realized how much fear I had carried in my body all those years, I nearly cried. My sorrow was more than just personal, it was for all the people who live in fear and bear the mark of it in every cell of their bodies.

Body stress is not always apparent

A lot of body stress goes unnoticed. It's like the background hum of white noise. We can get so accustomed to high levels of white noise that we don't hear the noise, and don't know it's affecting us and maybe even causing the headaches we get every time we go into a store or other building where the noise frequency is set especially high. (Did you know that some businesses even control the white-noise level this way to drown out other sounds that might distract you from doing business there?)

What tension or other physical distress are you feeling? Some of it may be obvious, some far less so. What if the stimulus for this distress disappeared? Would the distress also dissolve as it did in my case, or would it continue out of habit?

Sometimes we need to watch another person in order to help us recognize the imprint of mini-traumas on our own body. I attended a meeting of an association of personal coaches to learn more about this growing profession that helps people move forward with their personal and professional goals. The speaker that evening was Henry Kimsey-House, co-founder of the Coaches Training Institute. He demonstrated how he works with clients to help them get out of feeling "stuck." A local coach from the audience, a tall, slender, blond woman named Mary, came forward to volunteer as a client for the purposes of the demonstration.

In a flat, unemotional voice, Mary told Kimsey-House she loved coaching and was committed to being a great coach, but she hated having to market her business. She said that every time she had to face doing marketing activities, she froze up and couldn't do it. For her, the thought of marketing was traumatizing, and it was costing her a great deal emotionally and financially. She told Kimsey-House that she wanted to find greater ease with this necessary aspect of her business. He listened with full attention and compassionate eyes as she spoke, and then he responded, sometimes speaking directly to Mary and sometimes teaching the audience as he worked with her.

"Your face is getting squished up as you speak," he said to Mary in a gentle, nonjudgmental tone. He also pointed out to the audience that she was leaning forward—"trying hard, when what she wants is ease." As he made these comments, Mary smiled with obvious recognition and laughed. She sat back in her chair, and her facial expression softened. Just the recognition of how her body was holding this notion of marketing already began to decrease her stress. Still, she clearly wanted some resolution to her marketing dilemma. Kimsey-House asked her to talk more about her desire to be a "great coach." Mary became animated and her voice had a lilt to it as she spoke of how she loved helping people discover and pursue their passion. Kimsey-House noted to the audience that Mary had been "pressuring herself to market—something she hated," but that "*her energy* was in pursuing being a great coach." With that energy now ignited, Mary was smiling. Her shoulders were upright, her heart area was open, and her arms and hands moved with excitement as she talked. When Kimsey-House asked her how she felt about marketing at this point, she smiled widely, laughed an easy laugh, and declared, "I can do it."

While it represents a relatively minor trauma, this example illustrates well how mini-traumas that interfere with our daily life can be eased by first noticing their physical expression and then freeing the trapped energy beneath them. These mini-traumas may reflect more than the stressors of the moment. They may be reactivations of earlier trauma responses. Mary was probably reacting to more than the task of picking up a phone and making marketing calls. I know nothing of her personal history, but one possibility is that her "squished" face, her flat voice, and her forward-leaning "trying hard" were familiar manifestations of long-standing fears of failure, based on a string of harsh rejections in her past, perhaps beginning in childhood.

What would it feel like to have ideal parents?

Few of us had ideal parents. Our mothers and fathers and the other adults who were helping us made lots of mistakes. For many women, those mistakes left emotional scars that keep them "frozen," tense, or dysfunctional in other ways. One fascinating body-based form of therapy that addresses these early childhood traumas is Pesso Boyden System Psychomotor (PBSP). Clients in PBSP therapy who have painful childhood histories are helped to imagine an alternative upbringing, the kind that is in their best interests. This new version of the past is played out in a kind of elaborate therapeutic theatre that makes it seem emotionally real. The clients then have what PBSP therapists call a "virtual memory" of this more satisfying childhood to draw upon, which can be helpful in offsetting the long-term effects of early traumatic experiences. Creating alternative virtual memories can also work for traumatic events later in life.

Therapy based on body wisdom

The origin of PBSP was a series of exercises developed by professional dancers Albert Pesso and Diane Boyden-Pesso about fifty years ago. When teaching dance, they wanted to help their students tap into the emotional dynamics of their bodies so they could move with feeling. From these beginnings, the Pessos became deeply interested in the emotional scars carried in people's minds and bodies from past traumas, and they developed a way to help relieve people of these residual effects.

PBSP is highlighted in Maggie Scarf's book, *Secrets, Lies, Betrayals: How the Body Holds the Secrets of a Life, and How to Unlock Them.* Scarf talks about the many little traumas we experience in our lifetime that "leave their symptomatic calling cards." Everything from parents yelling at us as kids to a friend betraying us to the horrors of war bombarding us regularly from our TV screens can assault our sense of safety and well-being.

In response, our body, designed with inborn survival mechanisms, becomes hyperaroused—tense, ready for action—and hypervigilant, on the alert for danger. Or we "space out" and become emotionally distant in order to avoid what is too horrible to handle. Body tensions and illnesses develop and often persist. As Scarf put it when I met with her, "Even though we're not looking death in the face, we feel in danger, and our coping mechanisms are overwhelmed." The mind forms conclusions, often hidden from our awareness, such as "You can't trust anybody" or "I'd better just keep quiet." These thought patterns, too, register in our body.

In her book, Scarf cites PBSP as a powerful method for accessing these secrets the body carries by "summoning up a person's feelings, emotions, and sensations . . . during critical events or time periods of the individual's life." A therapy session, she says, creates "a taste of *what it would be like* to have had a different, more benign past and thus . . . engender[s] more hope-filled expectations that are rooted in the body."

Recast the past

In PBSP therapy, the physical activity and emotional display of the client are continually noted through "micro-tracking." This observation is done by someone playing the part of a "witness," a role-playing figure who names minute by minute what the client expresses in order to increase the client's awareness of her own physical and emotional state.

I had a chance to experience this process with Albert Pesso during an international PBSP conference. In my demonstration session with him, which took place in front of about forty observers, the witness was a symbolic figure, which Pesso placed in the air just above our heads. As I spoke or reacted, Pesso would say, "A witness would see how touched you are by that realization" or "From observing your sigh, a witness would see how relieved you are by that reassurance." I was often surprised as he named my reactions, which he would check for accuracy with me. I felt a degree of comfort, clarity, and intrigue, as if watching someone painting a true picture of me on canvas.

Pesso also noted any statements I made that sounded like dictums, such as, "I feel like I better get it right." He would say, "That sounds like a 'voice of truth,' so let's put that voice up *here* [pointing to another spot up in the air]: 'You better get it right.'" As he restated my words with the authoritative voice of a dictum, I could hear more clearly that this way of thinking was not mine but one imposed on me by my parents.

As my story emerged, I was soon crying, shaking, and curling into a hiding posture as I recalled some memories of harsh childhood experiences, mostly related to having to follow rigid rules that crushed my spirit. While I was in this state of freshly remembered trauma, Pesso helped me to develop another set of memories related to the original experiences. The goal was to help me become the "pilot" of my own life rather than to remain a trauma victim.

A major element in PBSP therapy is the client's assigning of roles to people or objects in the room to represent specific people or elements in the client's past. I chose a book to represent the rules from my childhood and a table as an altar to represent a strong church influence. Then I chose individuals in the room to represent specific family members as my story unfolded. In this drama, Pesso was helping me understand the "holes" my parents had in their own history that made it difficult for them to parent me well. I was also able to see the roles I had taken on to try to fill those holes, such as being a good girl to make life easier for my parents.

I assigned one person to play my dad as a boy, and then another pair of people to play his parents. As I saw how he had missed out on the nurturing and support he needed (because of his parents' holes), Pesso had me select another pair of people to play my dad's "ideal" parents. I gave them lines to say and actions to take toward my dad in his boyhood that were loving and encouraging. Watching this scene played out, I could believe that this boy would grow up to be a self-assured and loving father for me. In another scenario, I gave my mother an ideal husband so she could feel loved and supported, and wouldn't need me to fill that role.

Eventually, I picked two people to play my ideal parents. I had them stand behind me and, with reassuring touch and words, convey what I longed to hear as I was re-experiencing my childhood traumas. Using PBSP's therapeutic language, they said in unison, "If we had been your ideal parents, you would not have had to get things right. We would have loved you as you were. You would not have had to hide yourself from us. We would have been able to handle you."

As I heard these words spoken to me in a caring way and felt the message coming through in their touch, a huge sense of relief and freedom settled into my mind and body. Until playing out these scenarios, I hadn't realized how much I had hidden myself from my parents and from other people out of fear that I wouldn't be loved or would be a burden.

Having now *sensed* a possibility of having parents who were emotionally healthy and capable and who loved me unconditionally, I felt lighter and I started to laugh. I could feel what it was like to be enjoyed and supported by the adults responsible for caring for me as a child. Most important to me was the sense of being present in what felt like a village full of my ancestors, which I had been able to redesign as a healing, caring community into which I was then born. This very pleasant new memory is now implanted in my mind and body and gives me an ongoing sense of reassurance.

We shut down our feelings to stop the hurt

As Maggie Scarf points out and as the PBSP process reiterates, one common response to trauma is emotional shutdown, especially if the traumatic experience is continuous over a lengthy period of time. People affected by trauma "dissociate" or distance themselves from their feelings as a means of self-protection. It hurts too much to keep hurting so much; therefore, it seems better not to feel at all. Scarf writes in *Secrets, Lies, Betrayals*: "It is for this reason that children who've been severely stressed during their earliest years will so often grow up to become adults who are deaf to their own bodily cues and warning signals." A great many women endured some level of trauma when growing up, whether from witnessing their parents fighting, being bullied or rejected for being female or "fat" or "ugly," or experiencing some other form of abuse or neglect. Losing touch with their bodies became a way to hide out and feel a false sense of safety.

How in touch with your body are you? How aware are you of your body's distress signals?

Stop reading for a moment and observe what's happening in your body right now. Notice what your breath is doing. Observe any tension or effort you're making in your jaw and facial muscles, your neck and shoulders—anywhere in your body. Focus your attention on one of these areas of tension or effort. See if you can increase the effort. Then decrease it. Next, stop trying to change it. Just observe the effort your body is making in this area. Observe it closely for several minutes, noting any slight changes that occur as you pay attention.

Even if you've shut down your emotions and dissociated from your body because of a history of trauma, that doesn't mean your body is inactive. In fact, it's busy working to ensure your survival. Scarf says in *Secrets, Lies, Betrayals* that the body's "overall emergency warning system is on high alert and liable to be sounding off continually," prodding you to stay watchful for the ever-likely danger you fear. My body was in this state of emergency when I lived in the high-crime neighborhood. It was on high alert, with all the relevant body chemicals cued up for any necessary defensive action.

In her book, Scarf describes the effects of this perpetual high-alert status on a woman: "Although outwardly . . . responding calmly, her body is in a state of perennial readiness to meet with threat, and perfectly ordinary, neutral kinds of events can be experienced as catastrophic ordeals."

Mary, the woman in the coaching session with Henry Kimsey-House, appeared to be a calm and competent person overall, yet she was overreacting to the task of making marketing phone calls. I, too, am known for bearing a calm demeanor, but I used to experience frequent panic attacks. My body reacted as Scarf described—in the extreme—to challenges that were often as minor as having to decide how to organize my day. Intense and repeated childhood pressures to obey the rules and get things right made me highly fearful of making mistakes, creating a subtle traumatic imprint on my body that still gets activated at times when I try to meet expectations that are unrealistic.

Do you rarely relax? Do you overreact to mild challenges? Or are your emotions so dulled you feel little or no reaction at all, yet have physical problems you can't seem to clear up? Any of these conditions may be residuals of old trauma, or they may signal the existence of current mini-traumas you've become so accustomed to that you're blind to their effect on you. You may dismiss this state of affairs as normal stress, thinking "that's just life" and you have to "live with it." Not so. High-stress states are not normal—or necessary. Neither is living an emotionally flat existence.

As with major traumas (see chapter 4), you may benefit from the help of body-based counselors such as those who use drama or dance therapy techniques or PBSP. A bodyworker, body-awareness teacher, or personal coach can also open the way for fresh approaches to old problems through increased attention to your body's pleas for help.

A friend or circle of caring people can be another resource for you. The Focusing process described in chapter 4 can help relieve the effects of either major trauma or mini-traumas. It allows you to identify and name what you're feeling in the presence of loving witnesses who echo and validate your experience. The more you do this Focusing practice, the more you're likely to find your body eager to guide you to the kind of shifts you need to make.

EXERCISE: GET A WITNESS

Another approach is to ask your friend or group to note and describe your body language as you talk about a problem you're dealing with. Have them give you factual descriptions: "You're speaking very softly" or "Your fists clenched when you said that." In particular, ask them to tell you when they notice a change in your vocal tone, volume, and speed; facial expression and color; eye movements; hand movements; and posture. When they mention observing a change, bring your attention to that change as well. The changes are your body's way of revealing what's going on beneath the words.

Trust your body. Let it teach you. Don't try to stop or change what you're doing or feeling, but if the act of becoming aware of what your body is doing produces a change, follow that change and see where it leads. You may not get any big "aha" moments right away. Just observe and follow, trusting that your body wants to help solve the problem that is bothering you. It may take a while for you to find any significance in what's going on, especially if you've had little experience tuning in to your body's communication. As you notice certain body changes, you might be inclined to think, "I don't know what this means" and feel discouraged. Your task here is not to *know* in the intellectual sense, but rather in the somatic sense. Just stay attentive to what your body is doing in the present. Keep your focus there and be receptive to whatever happens. No *effort* is needed.

As you do this exercise, instruct your friends not to interpret what they see or to tell you what to make of it. Their task is simply to name what they see and hear. The goal is to help *you* become more aware of your body's communication. The more you are able to tune in to your body's expressions, the more you can discover what it wants you to know.

There are many variations to this exercise. You can ask your witnesses to point out anything that sounds like a "voice of truth" as you speak, as the therapist does in PBSP. Have them listen for expressions or statements you make that sound as if they might be coming from someone other than the grown-up you who is sitting there with them. These could be a vocal quality or a statement that sounds like a parent or a child. An example might be a strict-sounding "You should . . ." statement that is reminiscent of a demanding authority figure. Or it might be a childlike expression, such as a weak "I don't know what I'm supposed to do," accompanied by your shoulders shrugging. As you become aware of these different voices that direct your thinking, you'll notice that they are usually associated with some kind of body position, sound, or movement.

Listen to and dramatize your internal "voices"

You can expand this experiment to identify more of the various characters or roles that are part of the story you're telling. One day I was feeling extremely stressed by the load of too many projects to handle. My mind swirled with all the coming deadlines, calls to make, e-mails to send, and dozens of other tasks. I felt pressure on the sides of my head and tension throughout my arms, shoulders, and back. I was wearing out mentally and physically. Finally, it occurred to me to start listing out loud all the "voices" in my head that seemed to be weighing in on this problem. I noticed quite quickly that they all started with the words, "You should." *You should* be able to manage all this. *You should* be a lot more organized than you are. By this time in your life, *you should* be making a lot more money than you are, and then you wouldn't have to be doing all these things yourself. In no time, I had more than a dozen of these *shoulds* spewing out of my mouth. The clincher was, "*You shouldn't* be upset about any of this. None of these things are a big deal."

Well, there I was, upset from being at the mercy of all these *should* dictators and then being upset that I was upset. What chance did I have of getting out of this mess?

The first step was to recognize that I was not feeling stressed by the project to-do list itself. Rather, the *shoulds* filling my mind were creating the tension and distress I felt. I began to wonder: Where were these shoulds coming from? Who *says* that I should be more organized than I am or that I should make more money than I am? And how could I dethrone these dictators?

Each of these *shoulds* represented a voice that wasn't my authentic voice. (Who in their right mind would be so cruel to *herself!*) My next mission was to get acquainted with these voices as "roles" or "characters" that were still influencing me from past traumas and leaving me frightened, joyless, and ineffective.

How often do you find yourself in situations like mine where you're feeling pressured or tormented by some kind of internal conflict? Who might be the internal players in your drama? (Note: This is not a time to worry about how to deal with whoever was the original source of the "you should" messages or other pressuring statements. What's helpful here is to make the acquaintance of the disturbing voices or characters *inside yourself.* They, not the actions of others, are the real source of your distress now.)

Exercise: Inner Character Dialogue

There are many ways to meet, dialogue with, and reimagine these characters in order to reduce or redirect their influence on you.

One way to start is to say hello to them. The Buddhist teacher Thich Nhat Hanh suggests we welcome, rather than resist, our feelings. They are friendly messengers, wanting our attention. He says to greet them with "Hello, anger" or "Hello, fear" as they arise. If you find yourself feeling furious with your spouse or child because he left a pile of clothes or tools or toys right where you're likely to trip over them *again*, stop and welcome your response and make an effort to get acquainted with its plea. You might say, "Hello, anger. You're very big and fiery today. I'm eager to get to know you. Let's have a talk. I'm ready to listen and learn from you."

Since your feelings are reflected in your body, start to "listen and learn" by noticing how this anger is expressing itself in your body. Is your heart speeding? Do you feel any pressure anywhere in your head? Is there a surge of energy anyplace specific—or all over? Are your hands "burning" or stiffening or clenching? Do this observing without judgment (you are not *wrong* for feeling angry—nor right, for that matter) and with the sincere intention to appreciate how your anger wants to help. You are beginning the process of getting acquainted with this character or voice that is communicating with you.

Of course, you won't "hear" an audible spoken response, as you might when talking to another person. The response may come instead in the form of intensified body activities. Perhaps your fists clench tighter or your foot stomps. Or some image may come into your mind—let's say a fire or volcano. Or you might become aware of certain colors or sounds. Stay alert for whatever response, however subtle, you receive from welcoming your anger.

Continue the Inner Character Dialogue by acknowledging what you notice and expanding your welcome. "I can see your fire is even bigger than I realized. I'm glad you're showing it all to me." Or, "I'm enjoying the intensity of the red I see. I'd like to see more." After you make a comment or ask a question, pause, relax as much as possible, and open yourself to receiving a response. "Soften" your mind and body so you can be receptive to your imaginative, non-linear, wise inner workings.

If anything about the anger sounds, looks, or feels like someone you know from your past, you might ask if that is the "character" who has shown up in this anger: "You seem familiar to me. You remind me of my mother. Are you my mother's voice?"

You may have some intense emotional reactions as you take in the responses you're getting. Your mother's voice may be one you don't want to hear. Of course, the "voice" or "presence" that shows up is not the real person, but rather a legacy from that person, which you carry around inside yourself. So, it's really an aspect of yourself showing up. My *shoulds* are a good example. They represent old voices still broadcasting on my internal radio station. They reflect a traumatized part of me still in need of loving reassurance.

As you notice your reactions, you can add them to the dialogue, while continuing a friendly welcome: "I get scared when I hear your voice (the mother voice). I feel small and ashamed around you and want to hide, but because your voice is showing up inside me right now, I'm willing to get better acquainted with it."

You can continue this direct dialogue in a number of forms:

- Write the dialogue in your journal.
- Use pens, markers, chalk, or another art material to represent some part of the dialogue or the characters. Then look for themes that invite further dialogue or suggest courses of action.

- Imagine your anger or another internal "character" seated in a chair across from you. Speak your part of the dialogue aloud to this imagined person, feeling, idea, or object in the chair. Then move to the other chair, assuming the role of this character, and give a response.

- Role-play the dialogue in a full dramatic staging, giving an exaggerated voice and movement to each character, including the present "you," who is the prime player in the scenario.

- Include a wise, loving, compassionate God or other spiritual figures in the conversation. Ask for guidance or for mediation between the characters. Another option is to step into your own loving, compassionate, wise "higher self"—embracing the divine essence within you—to guide the conversation.

- Envision the "ideal" parents for this voice or character that is showing up, in a manner similar to what Albert Pesso does in his therapy sessions. Have another person, a pillow, or another object play the various roles, and give them appropriate lines and actions that result in the voice or character feeling completely accepted and unconditionally loved.

Play with paper "dolls"

One of the ways I engage in dialogue with various voices of distress that show up in my mind is with a set of homemade paper "doll" characters. One day when I was feeling particularly overwhelmed about how to manage all the various aspects of my life, I sat down with a set of watercolors and small strips of watercolor paper about the size of a large bookmark. I quickly—in a non-linear and free-association state of mind—painted each piece of paper with colors and freeform images that reflected one of the many opinionated entities that were vying for attention in my brain. Then I gave each of them a name. *Raja,* with red fireworks images, represented my anger. *Tiffany,* illustrated with washed-out cloudy shapes, was my timid, fearful, cautious side. *Sandy,* with the appearance of confetti on a bright yellow background, stood for my fun-loving, what-the-hell voice. *Love,* in a mix of yellow and red flames, was my loving nature. *Rosa*, looking like a set of square boxes, played the part of my financial manager.

I kept painting until I felt that all the points of view were represented—nineteen in all. I referred to these "people" collectively as my staff. I included a flowered *God* as my CEO. Then I bent a piece at the bottom of each strip of paper backward ninety degrees to create a base, so the paper could stand. I stood the paper characters in a semicircle and called a staff meeting. I asked "God" to moderate the conversation.

I have used this circle of paper dolls to sort things out and make decisions whenever I'm feeling distressed about something. I speak out loud in the role of each character. If I'm considering taking on a new activity, for example, Tiffany might say, "Well, I don't really know how to do that. I might get it wrong." Sandy would then laugh, retorting, "How bad can it get? We can just try it for a month. If we don't like it, we can stop. No harm done." Rosa would inject a word of caution, "I don't want to be a wet blanket, but we may lose a month of income if we back out after trying it out, and we can't afford that."

"God" encourages everyone at the meeting to voice their concerns and ideas, making sure everyone is heard. God also helps the group stay true to high spiritual ideals and serves as mediator when conflicts arise. So, at this point in the meeting, God might say, "Thank you, Tiffany, Sandy, and Rosa. Tiffany, I understand your reservations. If we decide to move ahead with this project, let's look at how to build in a way to help you learn whatever you need to feel confident. How does that sound? And Sandy, your go-get-'em attitude will be our inspiration if we get buy-in from everyone. Looks like we need to stay aware of the financial implications before deciding, though, as Rosa brought up. Does anyone else have something to say on this issue?" The dialogue continues until I and my "staff" come to some kind of resolution about the subject that's troubling me.

I have a lot of fun with this trauma drama. In a playful but direct way, I'm able to give voice to the various, and sometime conflicting, thoughts that have me in turmoil. "Hearing" and play-acting all these characters helps me not only to understand the diverse viewpoints tugging at my insides, but I am also able to feel the emotions behind the thoughts. Noticing the frightened, childlike sound of Tiffany's voice and feeling my body pull back in fear as I play that role helps me tune in to the unhealed aspects of the scared, traumatized child still living in me. Instead of trying to give in to or override this fear, as I might normally do while handling a challenging situation, I'm more inclined to create necessary reassurances for this scared little one. I do this reassuring through another one of the voices—often God or Love. The activity is similar to the "ideal parent" creation in PBSP.

From these staff meetings, I have also been able to discover many useful perspectives on troubling situations. Once I've given all the characters an understanding ear and any necessary reassurances, they usually become quite creative and cooperative in addressing the issue at hand. I'm often surprised by the new ways of thinking about the issue that I walk away with after these meetings. I'm more confident and comfortable regarding the issue because my inner turmoil has subsided considerably.

Alone, or with a small group of supportive witnesses, you can give voice to traumas that reside in your body through some type of physical expression. By doing so, the voices become a kind of separate entity from you, and you can discover ways to break their patterns or alter their effects on you.

What Does Your Body Have to Say?

OBSERVE AND REFLECT

DRAMA MAPPING: Identify a stressful situation you'd like to resolve. Draw a "map" of the players in the situations, with you as a circle at the center. Draw the other players as circles (or other shapes) positioned around you in a way that reflects their relationship to you and each other. Once you're satisfied that this map represents the situation and players adequately, stand in the center of the room you're in. Position different objects in the room around you in a way that mimics the drawing. Use an object to represent each person. If possible, have supportive friends stand in for some of the people. Then move around and observe the different "people" and their relationships. Reflect aloud on why you've arranged the people as you have and what you want from them.

You can also talk to certain people, move them around, stand "in their moccasins," or find other ways to physically engage with this live map of your situation. As you do, notice the reactions within your body.

The object of this activity is to help you gain insight into the situation that goes beyond just thinking about the situation. Your body knows what's needed, and if you tune in to its inclinations with curiosity, you may be surprised by what you'll experience and understand differently about the troubling situation. A sense of humor can also be quite helpful as you "direct" and play a part in this drama.

DRAMA ROLE-PLAYING: Make a list of body stresses you regularly feel. Choose one and make a list of your internal "voices" related to this area of stress that are competing for your attention. By yourself or with others who will support you, create a drama in which you act out each of the roles suggested by these voices. Step inside these roles as fully as you can, using gestures, tone of voice, or other expressions of these characters. Treat them with respect and genuine curiosity. They are a part of you. Let them have their voice, without censorship. In your dramatization, help them find a way to feel safe and secure. For example, a harsh, cursing voice may represent a person so frightened that he or she assumes the need to exert power abusively for self-protection. Play with ways to reassure and show compassion for this frightened part of yourself, so the need to exert power is lessened.

WRITE

DRAMA MAP WRITING: Journal about your observations in the map exercise above. Consider redrawing the map as your perceptions change or new ideas emerge.

WRITING IN YOUR DRAMATIC VOICES: In the second exercise above, allow each of the "voices" representing your body stresses to speak through writing.

IDEAL PARENT IMAGINATION: Write a few paragraphs, beginning with "When I imagine myself having ideal parents, I . . ."

LIVE

STOP AND OBSERVE: Do you find yourself overreacting to minor challenges? The next time you feel like hiding out or attacking in response to a perceived threat, stop yourself. Take a few conscious breaths and give your attention to your body's activities. Keep your attention on your body, even if your state of distress continues to mount. Observe the feelings and sensations in your body in the same way you observe dark clouds moving in across the sky, preparing to rain. Notice how they change over time. Eventually they will pass.

Notice if you're becoming more aware of your body as you read and do the exercises in this book. Is some of what's been "shut down" opening up a little?

CHAPTER 6

Relief for Bodies in Pain

We all hurt physically at one time or another. After a few decades of living, aches and pains seem to multiply and intensify. Major illnesses and diseases are more likely to show up. Some of this increase in symptoms comes from wear and tear, normal aging changes, health neglect, or genetic and environmental influences. Some of the body's mounting distress represents the persistent cries of unresolved traumas, a topic visited in the last two chapters. But some symptoms seem designed to increase our consciousness. They wake us up, prompting us to move toward deeper spiritual and emotional awareness in order to increase our overall well-being.

Awaken to self-damaging thoughts

One morning, as soon as my eyes opened, I felt engulfed in tension. Neck, shoulder, and arm muscles tightened. Forehead muscles scrunched. I lay there wishing I could find a delivery service for instant massage therapy.

My mind was racing too. Will I ever figure out the intricacies of my new computer? How will I pay off those monstrous medical bills? Oh no, I forgot to get oats for my morning oatmeal at the store yesterday—I'm going to go hungry this morning! And what about my trip this week to

Seattle and Vancouver and Victoria to give a series of talks and workshops? How will I ever get everything ready for that?

From past experience, I knew I was in trouble. Without decisive action, I could easily take a steep slide into depression or overeating or going out to spend money I didn't have!

I knew it was time to practice what I preach. Although my body and my mind were both radioing SOS, attempts at rational thinking weren't going to do the trick. At the moment, I couldn't trust my runaway mind as it rode the rails to imagined disaster. So I turned my attention to my body, which was the only "real" thing I could deal with. Aware that trying to "fix" my body's tension would do no good, I became curious instead. What *is* my body actually doing? What is it trying to say? Instead of trying to relax my muscles, I let them tighten all they wanted to. And they did.

My shoulders rolled inward and pushed upward toward my ears with full force, while my neck pulled downward and my arms pressed hard against my sides. Everything in my upper torso felt tight. What slowly became apparent as I experienced these tensions in volcanic intensity was that they were erupting out of two fears burning under the surface—the fear of not belonging (if I didn't prepare well enough, I'd be rejected by important others) and the fear of not surviving (unpaid bills and business failure = destitution = hunger/homelessness). In essence, I was afraid I might die or be abandoned. Pretty scary stuff! The body is designed to signal us when our basic needs for life and belonging appear to be in danger, and it was doing its duty well by me that morning.

By fully feeling the fear showing up in my body, I was honoring the messenger and welcoming its clues about what was wrong. No wonder my muscles tensed up, with all these frightening thoughts on my mind! It soon became very apparent that my irrational thoughts, not the current reality, was igniting my distress. At the moment, I was clearly alive (my body's activity was unmistakable evidence!). I was not being rejected by anyone (no one was anywhere in sight from my pillow view). I was merely lying in bed. Since the core fears of not living and not belonging were obviously based on false information, I decided to review my thinking that led to these primal reactions. Was I going to go hungry this morning? Not if I looked in the refrigerator and cupboard for other options. Were the medical bills going to go unpaid? Some might have to wait, but that's not a disaster and I'll have time to come up with more money. Will I be ready for my trip? I'll be ready as I can be, and that will have to be good enough. In the meantime, I can make a plan to get done what is needed.

As I adjusted my thinking, my body began to relax. I turned my attention to preparing for a workshop that I would give on my trip, and soon found myself excited about what I planned to teach. I was very glad that morning that I have a built-in feedback mechanism when my thinking runs amuck.

Who's got time?

But, you might say, I don't have the time to stop and listen every time I'm tense. I've got work to do, volunteer projects to manage, and my family always needs something. It would be easier to just pop one of my anti-anxiety pills, or take some kava kava and go on. Or if I just keep myself busy, my nerves will settle down after a while, or at least I won't notice the tension so much.

In my experience, listening to my body ends up saving me time. My body is my friend, looking out for my best interests. It tunes me in to reality. It's constantly making a record in my muscles and corpuscles of my thoughts and feelings, and throwing up red flags when I'm in self-damage mode. When I heed its call for attention, I am indeed slowed down, but if I settle into this slower mode, I can tune in better. What I've been hiding from comes into focus.

It's not *time* that keeps us out of touch with our body; it's timidity and momentum. We don't want to face that what we're doing isn't working. We want to do what we've always done, even if it's killing us. Strange, isn't it? We might even label it insane.

I notice this insanity most often when I'm working at my computer. My shoulder starts to hurt a little, then more and more—yet I push on. I'm eager to finish whatever I'm working on. Maybe I'm even enjoying the work. But my body is reporting that no, I can't keep working on it right then—at least not in the same way—without doing damage to myself. Something about the way I'm thinking (perhaps the need to "push" or the pressure I place on myself about a deadline) might be what's sparking the shoulder distress, or maybe my shoulder muscles just need relief from the repetitive pattern. If my mind isn't taking my body's well-being into account as part of the whole picture of getting the project done, then indeed I could be called insane—out of touch with reality.

EXERCISE: BODY CHECK-IN

A body check-in once an hour or so is a great way to stay present to my whole experience—to be *conscious*. You may wish to use this same body check-in practice for yourself when you're feeling tensions, headaches, or other signs of stress coming on—or, even better, as regular self-care *before* you start having any of these painful warning signs.

First, make a clear choice to give your body some time and attention for thirty seconds or more. Then, draw your mind away from its busy streams of thoughts and connect with your body. Make this connection by settling back in your chair and stroking your hands, thighs, or feet in order to direct your attention to your body. Some questions you could consider during a body check-in are: *Am I feeling relaxed and full of vitality? Or do I any feel any tightness, heaviness, restlessness, tiredness anywhere in my body? Do I feel as if I'm going to come apart? Is there a lot of adrenaline flowing? What does my body need at the moment? What areas of my body feel stable, at ease? What happens if I take some deep breaths? What if I drop my attention from my head (thoughts) to my heart (emotions) or to my belly (chi—the energy center)? What area of my body might beg for a stretch? What if I shake everything loose?*

A particularly good time to do frequent body check-ins is when you find yourself in situations in which your body has a history of developing painful responses. Let's say you often get headaches or a knot in your belly when you're around certain people. The more you consciously pay attention to your body's needs and signals, the more you'll pick up on "danger signs" in their early stages, before they become huge and perhaps develop into serious pain or illness. You'll also get reacquainted with how beautifully your body befriends you and how much smarter, healthier, and more "alive" you become when you honor that friendship.

Maybe now would be a good time to stop reading for a few minutes and check in with your body. If getting up and "shaking everything loose" feels like a good idea, do it!

Stay aware of changes that signal trouble

As you did the check-in, did you notice some familiar aches and tensions? Did you do what you usually do in the response to noticing them? Did it help? Sometimes health conditions become so familiar, we ease into resignation. Or we use a bandage approach, applying a little relief or cover for the symptoms while ignoring escalations or changes that need our attention.

A couple years ago, it took a dramatic turn of events to draw my attention to certain symptom changes in my own body that were quite serious. For several months, I had been experiencing rapid heartbeats fairly frequently. On the one hand, this didn't seem too out of the ordinary. A speedy heart, along with shortness of breath, was one of the symptoms of the panic attacks I'd had off and on for years. I had gotten used to these attacks and learned to deal with them as best I could. One of the most helpful strategies I had learned was to be very patient during an attack, knowing that it would eventually subside—in other words, not panicking over being in a state of panic.

So, when I felt shortness of breath and a rapid heartbeat as I went for an aerobic walk one Sunday, I did the usual thing. I slowed down, determining that I would take my time getting back home, where I would then relax as best as I could until the attack passed. However, the temperature outdoors was well below freezing that Sunday, and the more I walked (at my slowed pace), the colder I got and the faster my heart raced. I feared I would not make it back home without frostbite, if I made it at all.

I decided to stop in at an assisted living residence two blocks from my home, figuring I could warm up and slow my breathing down and then resume my walk home. The person at the front desk, seeing me in such a distraught state, was so alarmed that, over my objections, she called an ambulance. I was sure I could calm the symptoms myself in due time, yet my heart kept going faster, and I was hyperventilating at increasing intensity.

Still having great difficulty breathing and talking when the ambulance arrived, I told the technician that I was just having a panic attack and wanted to get home. She checked my pulse and heart and said that my heart rate was too fast for a panic attack. Worn down by my exhaustion and growing agony, I at last gave in and was whisked away to the hospital, where I kept cardiologists busy for several days, as they monitored my heart rate and poked around in my heart with catheters to fix what they called atrial flutter and atrial fibrillation. This was not a panic attack, they convinced me, but a set of errant patterns in my heart. It's possible that a panic attack set them off, the doctors said, though the cause of these patterns, in general, is uncertain. Maybe I'd never had panic attacks at all, one doctor strongly suggested. Maybe the irregular heart patterns had been the problem all along.

I don't know whether that doctor was right, but I learned many lessons from this experience. One of them is how, like most people, I tend to hold on to the familiar. I knew panic attacks. I had told stories about my attacks. I had written about them in familiar detail. Like many other people with chronic health conditions, I had incorporated my panic attacks as part of my identity.

Almost like a defiant child, I felt resistant to the new information the doctors were giving me. How could it be that what I had been so sure of was not the true story, or at least not the whole story? I had been experiencing a more erratic and insistent kind of rapid heartbeat in the past few months. That might explain it. Maybe this atrial problem was indeed new and had developed as the result of my history of panic attacks. Of course, I had ignored the recent observations about changes in my heartbeat, thinking they must be just another variation on panic attacks. After all, I had my identity story, and since this was one of the stories I'd claimed for myself, I tried to fit my present experience into what I already knew.

Once I had to face my own story and freshly re-examine it, I recognized that when I become so "sure" of something, I may miss what my body is saying in the present because I'm caught in a past story. Humbling. Amusing, too. How funny that we humans love our stories so much, even our painful ones, that we hate to give them up.

Avoid doing a rush job on yourself

My hospital experience taught me another important lesson about familiar patterns. Like a lot of people today, I tend to live life as if everything is *urgent*. Life is moving fast, and I have to keep up. I can easily justify this rushing because of my "busy" life. I think I'm being efficient by moving quickly and multitasking. Sometimes all this speed and busyness results in a lot of tension, but I'm usually quick to reassure myself that I'm all right because I know how to de-stress from time to time.

After four hospital stays slowed my pace dramatically, I got another sense of time altogether. For weeks, medication side effects and pain levels (from procedural complications) made it necessary for me to move at an unfamiliar slow pace, concentrating on just one thing at a time, completing one thing before starting another, and taking a rest between activities. To my surprise, I began to like this pace. I was doing things with a greater sense of ease. I enjoyed the sense of mindfulness I was experiencing. I wasn't getting tense.

I did worry at times that the items on my to-do list wouldn't get handled. Yet in my mindful state, I began to notice that most things *were* actually getting done, with more ease than usual. I began to wonder: could it be that it's not necessary to race at such high speed? Maybe I'd actually get more done if I operated at a slower speed. It didn't sound reasonable, but it felt good.

As my physical strength and my ability to think clearly returned to normal, I paid close attention to the speed of my activities. One day I noticed myself grabbing my keys and rushing to get in my car. How silly it seemed to be rushing. What was the rush anyway? All the rushing around was doing was creating tension. I wasn't really getting things done faster, because in my rush I'd tend to forget or drop things. I was learning that slower feels better and gets faster results. That may not be logical, but it's real.

What about you? Are you taking the time you need for your own well-being? Or is the pressure of the clock running your life? Loving attention to your body will help to answer that question.

The more we live with conscious awareness of our body, the more quickly we're able to notice pain in its earliest stages and respond with appropriate measures to learn from it and alleviate it. Most often the ailments we experience have been trying to get our attention long before we notice them.

Trust the "force of silence"

Arnold Mindell, the brilliant visionary and psychotherapist who weaves together bodywork, Jungian therapy, quantum physics, and more, talks about paying such close attention to our body that we notice the subtle tendencies to activity that exist before we actually move. In *The Quantum Mind and Healing: How to Listen and Respond to Your Body Symptoms,* he suggests that there is an inclination, a kind of primal force—he calls it the "force of silence"—that drives our movement. Mindell talks about this force as quantum waves and uses other terms from physics that I can't quite follow. My simple term for what he is talking about is "impulses." They are promptings that try to move us toward a state of well-being. They reflect not only our personal history and mythology but also community and universal influences. If unheeded, they can become precursors to illness and disease.

Mindell says that these impulses—this force of silence—is key to understanding ourselves and our world. "To use this force—to learn to move with it and work with symptoms—you need only to learn to focus your awareness during stillness," he writes. This is not a mental state of awareness, but a more dreamlike state—what might be described as *being* rather than *thinking about.* We can be so *present* to our body experience, for example, so absorbed in what is going on without having any agenda but attentiveness, that a shift in our state of health occurs without any conscious effort. In the introduction to this book, I described how long-standing tension in my neck dissipated as I sank into absorbed attention. Allowing my neck to follow impulses toward movement eventually freed me to "hang out" in a state of ease rather than push my way through life in my usual mode.

Mindell doesn't discount the biomedical perspective on illness, nor do I. He offers an alternative window into our symptoms: "You are having big dreams in your body and (in a way) are lucky to receive dramatic messages from the force of silence." He calls chronic symptoms "koans," which he describes as "apparently unanswerable questions meant to increase our consciousness."

What are the "big dreams" in your body? What questions are your symptoms prompting you to consider? You don't need to come up with definitive answers for these questions. You can just *be* with them. They are not mind exercises. Let your body *live* into the answers, offering you inner promptings that reflect a knowing that goes beyond thought.

Mindell even offers a bold vision of a doctor's visit in an ideal future medical model that incorporates this added way of appreciating the body's wisdom. The doctor invites the patient to become fascinated by the presenting symptom and, like a Zen master, poses a question to prompt the patient's self-exploration. The doctor in this scenario might even offer the patient guidance—something like this, says Mindell: "Your symptoms of fatigue and persistent aches and chest pressure are the beginnings of a dance. Let your body dance and express whatever is in your chest creating that pressure." Dance that comes from such intrinsic impulses gives expression to what wants to be healed. The force of silence has its say, choreographing our moves through our symptoms toward wellness. Personally, I long for the day when doctors routinely become our guides to self-healing body awareness.

Steep yourself in the now

Like Mindell, Eckhart Tolle recommends stillness or silencing of the mind in order to address what he calls the "pain-body." While it's normal for emotions to come and go quickly, explains Tolle in *The Power of Now*, "when you are not in your body, an emotion can survive inside you for days or weeks." When more than one emotion takes up such a lengthy residence, the multiple emotions can combine and become "the pain-body, a parasite that can live inside you for years, feed on your energy, lead to physical illness, and make your life miserable." In other words, as he explains in an interview with *Science of Mind*, negative emotions that are not fully acknowledged and accepted stick around, leaving "a residue of emotional pain, which is stored in the cells of the body."

Tolle's invitation is to watch our pain-body silently, not with the mind but by directing our attention to what Tolle calls the "inner body" or the "subtle energy field that pervades the entire body and gives vibrant life to every organ and every cell."

See if you can feel this inner body or field of energy that Tolle describes now. It is not your physical body, but rather the experience of yourself deep inside and around your body. If you try to *think* your way into finding it, it will elude you. Instead, let yourself *feel* the pulsation of life that runs through you. As you experience this vibrancy, you will be in the state of being that bridges your physical form and your deepest spiritual essence. You will be, as Tolle says, in the *now*.

From this keenly present experience within your inner body, observe an area of discomfort—your pain-body. Watch it without identifying with it. It is as if you are stepping back and watching this person who is you having this experience of pain. Time stops. You are the disinterested, dispassionate watcher. You are not looking to accomplish anything, not even a change in the pain. If resistance or other mind chatter shows up, you watch that also, accepting whatever arrives without identifying with it. Stay in the now, in the realm of the inner body, in stillness.

Notice that your conscious attention, if sustained, has a transmuting effect. The mind plagued with negative emotions, claiming justification for holding onto resentments or succumbing as victim to surrounding threats, loses its grip. The emotions dissolve. And the body chemistry shifts accordingly.

You may not experience a full shift of this kind the first time, or even the second or third time you step into the *now* experience. You may just feel a hint of it. Maybe a little of your tension or pain diminishes, or you have a sharper sense of hearing or seeing. Let each experience of being in your inner body—in the *now*—help you feel more at home in your body. At the same time, know that you are more than your body. The *now* experience opens your awareness to the divine life force pulsing through you, which is always directing you toward a state of wellness.

Claim your divine health

Stillness was the entryway to health for Myrtle Fillmore, the early twentieth-century pioneer in fostering the mind-body-spirit connection. For Fillmore, "going into the silence" was a frequent practice she used to open herself to the influence of God. It was under this influence that she evolved from being a self-described "emaciated little woman" into a vibrantly healthy woman who lived to the age of eighty-six. "In seeking health," she writes in *Myrtle Fillmore's Healing Letters*, "we are to pray for an understanding of our oneness with God, to claim it." "Claim it" is the key phrase here. She assumed that the life—the substance—of God is within us, and that includes perfect health.

When we experience pain or sickness, she says, we have "lost track of our hold on the gifts of God." The path to health, according to this advocate of practical spirituality, is to reclaim our alignment with God or, more specifically, the divine life flowing through us. Fillmore adamantly subscribed to a statement she had heard from a preacher as a young woman, when she was plagued with life-threatening tuberculosis and other serious conditions: "I am a child of God, and I do not inherit sickness." This statement so startled her when she first heard it that it completely changed her way of thinking—and eventually her state of health. She began to keep her mind focused on God and on her divine inheritance expressed in every cell of her body. To put it simply, she "listened" for the *health* in her body, believing deeply in her body's perfect functioning until this health showed up in physical form.

Myrtle Fillmore talks about this process in her writings, inviting us to "re-educate" our thoughts to hold a spiritual image of our body as healthy, *despite appearances*. She is not suggesting that we ignore what hurts or that we neglect appropriate care. But she is suggesting that we deny illness the ultimate power in our life and give our primary attention to spiritual practices and thoughts that have the power to rearrange the cellular activity of the body. Keeping this perspective is important, she says, because "our body temple is the fruit of our mind."

This change in physical health takes more than just positive thoughts, however. It's part of a whole program of deep self-listening and action directed toward our overall well-being. Fillmore says (using the archaic, male-dominated language of her era) that a person who aligns with "God-mind" and holds thoughts of bodily perfection also "looks into all his thought habits to see that they are prompted by faith and divine love and wisdom and life and joy and freedom." She is calling for a complete mental, emotional, and spiritual makeover.

But she doesn't stop there. Arranging your living habits so that your body is well cared for is also part of this path to healing. The person on this path, she writes, "acquaints himself with the different parts of the body, and learns what it is they are truly built for. He learns what each needs and supplies them." The final part of Fillmore's plan for creating health is declaring through affirmative prayer the "Truth" of our body's divine inheritance of health. This type of prayer is not a plea for healing but a statement that assumes the divine presence is at work in the body and the physical manifestation of that healing is now taking place. Fillmore's simple wisdom, when packaged as a whole, offers a full course in forming a healing mind-body-spirit connection.

When I first read Fillmore's works some years ago, I decided to test out her approach. I had sprained my left thumb in a fall, and because I used it so much in my everyday life and occasionally aggravated the injury, my thumb kept hurting for months. With Fillmore's guidance in mind, I invoked the "Truth" of God's perfect life within me. I visualized my thumb as working beautifully, consistently holding in my mind images of myself typing, playing tennis, digging in my garden, and doing other favorite activities with ease. I stopped thinking of my thumb as a "problem" and celebrated God at work in my body, especially in my thumb. During this time, I did my best to keep my thoughts in alignment with God throughout the day. I also took extra good care of my thumb and spoke words of love and appreciation to it. Within a very short time, the pain in my thumb was gone. I have seen many other people apply this process to heal from major health challenges, ranging from disabling car accident injuries to cancer.

If you have a persistent health problem, try a similar approach yourself, using these steps as a general guide:

- Make the commitment to align yourself with God or whatever you consider your spiritual Source.

- Review your thoughts that are wedded to fear, failure, or smallness, and let them go.

- Bathe your body in the experience of being one with your Source. Know yourself as the expression or extension of your Source.

- Claim your inheritance as a beloved child of the universe. Give thanks to your divine Source for vibrating through the cells of your body, giving you life and health. Thank your body for being a welcoming home for divine life.

- Imagine your body, especially the challenging area, operating with ease, doing the things you most love to do.

- Be kind to your body. Tend to its needs in a loving manner but don't dwell on the pain or discomfort. Turn your attention to thinking of your body as filled with revitalizing energy, functioning perfectly.

- Declare repeatedly, with conviction and feeling, a life-giving affirmation such as "I am the radiant life of God" or "I am vibrantly healthy in mind, body, and spirit."

- Continue this practice daily. Stay alert for changes in your physical, mental, and spiritual well-being.

Listen for your own awakening

Your aches and pains can lead you to expanded consciousness. They can help you discover ways that you contribute to your own ill health. They can bring you into closer touch with the spiritual dimensions of your life. They can coax you to make healthy changes in your life.

As you try some of the approaches described in this chapter, do so with an open, curious mind. They are not formulas but rather invitations to expand your self-knowledge and sense of well-being. They may cure your body, or they may show you a more enriching way to live with your health challenges. Listen and learn. Be still and wake up.

When you don't get better

When you understand the role you play in your own health, it can be easy to slip into discouragement or feelings of guilt when your health problems remain despite your best efforts to heal them: *What's wrong with me that I created such problems for myself? How come I'm not getting better, with all the spiritual insights I have?* More helpful questions might be: *What can*

I create in this situation that will serve my highest good? What is this illness calling me to become?

I witnessed a transformation in one of my sisters, a Catholic nun who went by the name Sister Patricia Ann, as she lay dying from cancer at the age of fifty-one. Despite the top-notch medical treatments she received, the loving care and prayers of the nuns around her, and her own heroic efforts to be healthy, she still suffered through the lengthy, agonizing decline of her health and finally death. Sister Pat, as I called her, was thirteen years older than me and had a major hand in raising me in my early years before she left for the convent. We shared the same wide smile, small eyes, and tall frame. Our laughter and speech patterns, too, were alike. In our adult years, I was sometimes ill at ease around her firm-set jaw, controlling personality, and driven nature that had helped to shape much of what I disliked in myself.

Her illness stripped away all that. As she lost control of her body—and of most everything—and came to rely on the care of others, she learned to love with her whole heart. Toward the end of her life, she had come to a point of surrender, savoring a deep sense of union with God that perhaps she could not have accessed without the experience of intense suffering. In her journal, she wrote, "My being is filled with an inner joy today though the body aches on . . . the love I feel flowing in me is so soothing; it has a healing power that transcends pain." Perhaps illness is our invitation to transcendence. Sometimes that transcendent state results in physical relief. Sometimes it lifts us beyond concern about pain to what really matters. Either way, I'd called that healing.

What Does Your Body Have to Say?

OBSERVE AND REFLECT

LESSONS FROM PAIN: Think about an illness or experience of pain you've had. What has that condition taught you? How do you see your life differently because of it?

NOTICE YOUR PACE: Pay attention to how fast you're moving through your days. Are you moving at the actual speed of life or at a speed invented by your mind? How does your body's health reflect your pace?

PAIN BENEFITS: Ask yourself what you get out of having the pains and illnesses you have.

BODY CHECK-IN THOUGHT CHANGING: For one whole day, set a timer to go off every hour. When the timer goes off, take a minute or so to do a body check-in. Each time, thank your body for its signals of distress or well-being. Make a note of any thoughts that might be triggering whatever distress you are feeling. Change them, if you can easily do so, in the moment. If you have trouble changing them on the spot, set aside a time at the end of the day to examine your thinking more fully and make adjustments.

WRITE

REFLECTIVE JOURNALING: Journal as a way to reflect further on the above activities.

CHANGING THE "INSANE": Plan to spend at least a half hour on the following exercise. Make three columns on a piece of paper. In column one, list any mindsets or behaviors you have that are "insane," in conflict with reality. Examples might range from smoking to holding onto resentments to working too many hours. For each one, note in column two the physical, emotional, and spiritual price you pay for maintaining this mindset or behavior. If you're not sure, become still and ask your body to help you grasp what this issue is costing you. In column three, for each item reflect on what it would take to stop hurting yourself this way. Saying a prayer or spending time in silence may help you determine what you could do differently. Put one word, phrase, or image in column three to represent this action. Let your entries in the third column be your guide for a week and record the results in your journal.

LIVE

AWARENESS IN THE SPACES: In your day-to-day life, experience the space between your thoughts, just as you experience the gaps between sounds in music that allow you to hear the notes. In those time spaces, slip into awareness of your inner body. Experience the *now*.

CHAPTER 7

Addictions: What Do You *Have* to Have?

What are those things you're always doing that you know you need to stop? You know the kind—the secret habits that mess up your life and leave you feeling ashamed. This chapter invites you to step into freedom by facing and stopping these self-destructive behaviors. Looking honestly at them may seem scary at first. Yet if you don't address these habits—which could be called addictions—they may eventually kill you, spiritually, emotionally, and physically.

This may be the most important chapter in the book for you, especially if your life is feeling out of control. It may help you get to the bottom of what's blocking your peace of mind. It may start to free you from what's running your life and from your shame about it. (If you're pretty sure that you don't have self-destructive habits and your life is going fabulously, I invite you to read this chapter anyway. Use it as a guide to help you understand your friends or family members who are struggling with addictive habits.)

Of course, facing your secrets means facing the truth. It takes courage to be honest. Perhaps more importantly, it takes compassion to keep from judging yourself. Women are so conditioned to feel shame. We have been viewed for so long as "less than," "dumb," "ditzy," "highly emotional, "conniving," and even "sluts" that we can easily sink into self-condemnation. We may feel like failures, unworthy, hopeless. The moment we recognize something less than ideal in ourselves, it becomes one more cause for self-flagellation.

In looking at your self-destructive behaviors, it's very important to be kind to yourself. You will be facing the truth, all right, but a big part of that truth is that you've done the very best you could with what you know so far. You've made choices that seemed in your best interest at the time. No one can do any better than that. You're not wrong or bad. You have not failed. You've lived what you learned and now, with the wise guidance of your body, you can learn something that will serve you better. Just as you've so often gently and compassionately helped children, friends, and others grow and make changes in their lives—without judging them—treat yourself with that same respect and gentleness as you face the truth and prepare to change. Easy does it. One step, one day, at a time.

What are you doing with your time?

Jenny wants to get back to work *now*. She's having lunch with a good friend at a neighborhood cafe, and she smiles and nods as her friend speaks. But her mind is mainly elsewhere. She's calculating how soon she can politely make an excuse to leave. Talking with her friend is nice, she thinks, but she can't wait to get back to that new project she's taken on at work. Besides, she has a ton of e-mails to deal with. Her friend invites her to go to a play with her this weekend. It's a play Jenny would love to see, but she says no, she has to work all weekend. The business she's developing on the side takes all her spare time. In fact, Jenny was up until after midnight last night working on it, so she's tired and has a hard time even listening to her friend. Still, her mind is busy. She's coming up with another twist for the new business, tuning out what her friend is saying about a book she just read.

Jenny is addicted to work. It's running her mind, exhausting her, and throwing her life completely out of balance.

Denise's greatest love in life is food. The refrigerator and the cupboards are on her mind more than anyone or anything else in her home. How much ice cream is left in the container and when can she justify having the next bowl of it? How many of the chips can she eat and still have some left so her husband doesn't complain again that she's eaten half the bag? A half hour after breakfast, she begins watching the clock. She doesn't plan to eat until noon, but would it hurt anything to have a few bites of something around ten o'clock, or maybe at nine-thirty before she gets too busy? In fact, maybe she'll bake some cookies—for the grandkids. Oh heck, the leftover popcorn from the night before on the counter should be eaten up, so the bowl can be washed. Her thinking continues like that all day.

Denise is a food addict. She often eats in secret and feels deep shame about her weak will and the size of her body.

Most of us crave *something,* one thing that we turn to religiously to give us a major boost—a kind of "high." For some of us, this craving is relatively harmless. We find a real delight in routinely knitting, playing tennis, or watching a favorite TV show. For many of us, though, what we crave becomes so central to our life that we feel sure we just can't do without it. If it's not available *when we want it,* we start to obsess about it, becoming almost frantic. When it appears out of reach, it's on our mind almost constantly. We feel as if our life is greatly out of sync until we have this *something* that we consider essential. Even the seemingly benign activity of knitting can become like a drug if it's used to "calm our nerves" and we feel anxious until we can get our hands on our needles again.

Check this out for yourself. If you couldn't have the following things *when you wanted them,* is there one or more of them that would you feel extremely upset about missing?

Your morning coffee?
Chocolate?
Time at the casino?
Your particular seat at the breakfast table?
Shopping?
Wine, beer, or spirits?
A round of golf?
Sex?
Your workout program?
Your work?
Approval?

Maybe your *something* isn't on this list. But chances are you've got one. Most women I've talked to, when they're really honest, admit to being compulsive about something. Take a mental inventory of the frequent activities in your day or week to see if there's something you think you can't manage without (not counting your loved ones and your basic needs)—something you're very attached to and that you make lots of effort to ensure you'll have available when you want it. An even bigger clue than your thoughts about this indispensable *something* is your bodily reaction when you're aware you might not be able to have it. In your thoughts, you can rationalize that work or golf or a casino trip is a good thing and that it makes sense to feel disappointed if you can't get to it. But your body will quickly tell you if what you value has gone from being a pleasant part of your life to being an uncontrollable, and perhaps self-destructive, craving. If you imagine being without that desired *something* at a time when you want it badly, notice if you feel a tightness in your belly, a headache, shaking, restlessness, irritability, or some other physical sense of urgency or pressure that has a desperate quality to it. These are signs not of normal disappointment, but of addiction.

You may be thinking: *What's wrong with enjoying life a little—having something that makes you feel good? Coffee and shopping—they make my day. And what is approval doing on the list? That's no "addiction." Everybody wants approval.*

Good feelings are one thing. Irrational, out-of-control cravings are another. I'm not talking about an occasional glass of wine or trip to Macy's with a friend. I'm referring to whatever gets you seriously bent out of shape when it's calling to you and you can't have it. Are you consuming liquor in large quantities? Often? In hiding? And then counting the hours or minutes until the next drink? Are you spending much of your spare time on eBay looking for bargains and accumulating closets full of things you never use? Some out-of-control cravings or addictions have obvious, serious consequences. Too much caffeine can harm your health. Compulsive gambling, drinking, and spending often lead to financial and family ruin, among other disasters. Some addictions have less obvious but still significant and costly effects. An obsession with watching TV may cloud out needed attention to work, family, or other major responsibilities. It may also create a distorted sense of reality. People who work compulsively can get a false sense of personal worth from their jobs, and neglect their health and important personal relationships.

For many women, approval is addictive. They build their lives around getting people to like them, not around what fulfills them or makes them happy.

Marlene learned early in life to get approval by taking care of other people. Over time, her need to fix other people's problems so dominated her life that, by her fifties, she often felt alienated from her authentic self. In public, she always wore a smile, cheered people up, and rushed to the rescue anytime someone seemed in need. Friends and family could count on her to show up if they were sick, needed a ride somewhere, or had a volunteer project in need of workers. Marlene's co-workers relied on her to fill in for them, find resources they hadn't gotten around to finding on their own, and lend an ear when they'd been wronged. Marlene was there for everyone but herself. She was well-liked and got the approval she worked so hard to get with her "good" behavior.

Yet this approval was a poor substitute for the unconditional love she wanted more than anything. She wanted to be accepted, whether she was on good behavior or not, even in her most scared, lonely, and selfish moments. But by always showing up in her high-spirited rescue mode, she only got what she set people up to give her—approval for her helpfulness. The real Marlene remained largely hidden from others and from herself. Because she spent enormous energy putting up this false front and working on others' behalf, Marlene was frequently tired. When she needed help herself, she was reluctant to ask for it and didn't think she deserved it. Instead, she would make the effort to help someone else, seeking once again the familiar kind of false love in response.

Addiction may seem like a harsh word to use for such behavior. But calling compulsive behaviors "addictive" is not meant to induce shame. Instead, the purpose is to draw attention to what takes you away from your *self* and your spiritual Source, and to invite you back home. Addiction is a form of worship. When you devoutly and consistently give your will and your life over to large amounts of tranquilizers, food, shopping, work, someone else's opinion, or anything else outside yourself in order to feel happy, it becomes your god. If you have addictive tendencies, you keep wanting more of this *something*. Yet the more you get of this illusive deity, the less satisfied you are. The cravings intensify mercilessly. You become a slave to their demands.

These addictive patterns register in your body. Your cravings and your response to them influence your nervous system, blood flow, metabolism, posture—your entire physical system. You may feel an adrenaline rush, nervousness, or an endorphin high. Your blood pressure may spike or your stomach could be in knots.

Marlene wanted to stop her cycle of approval-seeking. A deeply spiritual woman, her desire was to extend kindness out of genuine love rather than engage in approval-seeking rescue missions. But her craving for approval had so dominated her thinking and behavior that she no longer felt sure of the difference between these two modes of operating. (This often happens with addiction, losing a sense of what's genuine or normal.)

I invited Marlene to quiet her mind and check in with her body in order to observe these two modes. I watched as she first recalled a time when she was kind in order to get approval. Her facial muscles tightened. Her head jutted slightly forward. Her shoulders rolled inward. Her hands lifted slightly off her lap. It was as if she were moving ahead of herself, leaving herself behind to grasp for this "fix." "Oh yeah, I feel like I *have* to do this," she said, recognizing her familiar state of anxious compulsion to help. Then I asked Marlene to recall an experience of just *being* with someone—open, loving, and available—without the need to fix anything. Her face softened. She sat back in her chair, her shoulders drawn back and downward. Her hands relaxed on her lap. Tears came, as they often did whenever Marlene came to a moment of spiritual truth for herself. "I could feel the difference," she said, excitedly. "When I love people instead of grasp for their approval, it's easier. I'm not trying to get anything from them. And I'll bet I don't confuse people." In this moment, Marlene was breaking her pattern of addiction to approval. By learning from her body, she was taking small steps to end the confusion and distortion she felt inside herself and that she communicated to others.

How much of your day do you spend *going out of your way* to get someone to like you or think of you as a good person? How does this feel in your body? Can you recognize the difference in your breath, muscle tension, digestion, and energy when you help someone from the fullness of your heart instead of from a need to "be nice," "look good," or "give in"?

Fill up on what counts

Food is another common area of obsession for women. Consider the alarming upsurge in obesity that has medical experts greatly concerned these days. At the same time, anorexia and bulimia in young women are rampant, and most women's magazines and websites virtually shout "diet" like a loud mantra from their pages. Clearly, food is on women's minds a lot. For many women, obsessing about food, dieting, and body image fills hours of their time every day. For others, the preoccupation with food is more subtle, like steady background music they're barely aware of but that influences their mood.

By itself, food is emotionally neutral. But of course we like our eating experiences to be pleasurable. We choose foods that taste good, and our eating can be a highly sensual and socially satisfying experience. Think of the most savory soup you've ever tasted or the lunches you enjoy with good friends. In addition, preparing meals can bring out our creativity and be a way to show love to the people who matter to us. Food can indeed be a source of healthy and natural pleasure.

When does food become dangerous? When it becomes a substitute for what you really need or want.

Denise, the woman at the beginning of the chapter whose thoughts focus on the refrigerator, works in her own home business. She spends much of her day alone, communicating mostly by e-mail. She is overweight, and her cupboards hold a supply of diet products from several weight loss programs she has tried. Her marriage is shaky, and she worries about having enough money, especially if she ends up divorced. Denise is often hungry, but not for food.

Denise eats when she feels restless, has computer problems, thinks about her marriage, fails to get a customer she wants, feels lonely, has a crabby customer. She eats when it's a rainy day. She eats when she has too much to do and when she has nothing to do. Denise also eats when she has a headache, when her legs hurt, and when something she just ate didn't taste very good. After each meal, she eats "just one more thing." Her first thought, whenever she feels any kind of discomfort or even when she's feeling elated, is to reach for something from the kitchen to tame that feeling. Denise is afraid to feel, and afraid to deal with the issues underlying her feelings. Her emotion-numbing "drug" of choice is food.

Denise's case may be extreme, but her way of dealing with her emotions is all too common. Plenty of women dive into chocolate or chips or pretzels—or even gourmet meals—to give themselves brief moments of pleasure that will hide them from the rest of their lives. They literally lose themselves in food. After a while, the true pleasure of eating disappears, and only the idea of "more" drives them to the kitchen—*again.*

This compulsive eating mode is sometimes replaced with a drive to diet. Then, food becomes the enemy and discipline the god. The rationales for various diets and eating programs are myriad. Few of these approaches lead to successful weight management, and even fewer to peace of mind.

What is your relationship with food? When and how often do you eat? How much of the time are you eating in a way that honors your body?

What does your body really want and need?

When your body is hungry, it will send you a very clear signal. Your stomach feels empty. That's the most emphatic sign of hunger. Your stomach may even growl to make the message extra clear. Your energy level can also seem a bit low, and you may lose some mental clarity. These are the signs of ordinary hunger (not the desperate hunger of the starving). It seems elementary to list them, but because so many of us have a distorted sense of being hungry, it also seems important to reestablish what's normal.

So many of our modern eating habits overall are outside the norm. Eating on the run whenever we can squeeze it in. Eating foods that aren't satisfying for more than a few minutes. Eating sweet, salty, fatty foods because they're cheap and handy.

As we age, our body becomes less tolerant of unhealthy foods. The cumulative effect of eating them may be the emergence of diseases and disorders that force us onto restricted diets. Diabetics have to monitor nearly every morsel they put in their mouths and have to depend on more than hunger to give them clues about when they need to eat. Heart patients may have to limit certain fats and salt. Food sensitivities make eating out almost impossible for some women.

Yet the cravings continue because our most genuine hungers remain unsatisfied.

Denise craves companionship and a sense of safety and security. She longs to be touched affectionately. She wants to work with people she enjoys and to feel that her contributions are valued. She has many wants and needs. In any given moment, her addictive "habit" of turning to food (or concentrating on dieting) obscures these wants and needs, along with her feelings about them.

Mindful attention to her body and to the use of food can help restore Denise to sanity—to her*self!* It can do the same for you, if you have unhealthy ways of dealing with food. Becoming aware of how, when, and what you eat can help you address what's eating you, so you stop using food as a substitute for living.

EXERCISE: FOOD AND FEELING DIARY

The first way to approach this mindfulness process is by paying close attention to what happens when you eat. For three days, keep an honest and complete record each time you eat. Write down what you ate and the time you ate it. Also record the thoughts and feelings you had before you ate, as well as your body state. Finally, make note of how satisfying this eating experience was for you.

To prepare this log, take a sheet of paper and, across the top, write the five headings below. Enter the relevant information in the column under each heading whenever you eat.

Food/drink	Time of Day	Thoughts Feelings	Body State	Level of Satisfaction

Be specific in your record keeping. List *everything* you eat and drink, even if it's just one chip or raisin. In noting your thoughts and feelings, identify briefly their cause: "scared I'll run out of money this month," "disgusted with myself that I'm not doing as well as Jane," "angry that Ted didn't call today," "unsure about whether or not I should quit my job," "I really shouldn't have two cookies." You may have too many thoughts and feelings to record them all. Record those that stand out as particularly prominent. If your thoughts and feelings aren't very clear, just do the best you can.

Under the "Body State" heading, jot down whatever you can recall was happening in your body prior to eating: "tense in my shoulders," "fingers swollen and in pain," "eyestrain," "fidgety," "sleepy." Note anything at all that felt uncomfortable, even the feeling of hunger itself. Ideally, do a body scan to notice your body state *before* you begin eating. In the final column, rate your overall level of satisfaction with your eating experience, based on how nourishing and tasty the food was, how much enjoyment you felt while eating, how your body reacted to the food, and how much you ate. In other words, is this an experience you'd like to repeat? Rate your experience on a scale of one to five—a five if the overall eating experience was very satisfying, a one if it was lousy.

Don't make any big changes in your eating during these three days. Think of yourself as a scientist doing an objective case study of one person's way of dealing with food. You are simply observing and noting on paper your eating-related activities. Avoid any judgments during this period. Self-criticism is a setup for discouragement and for abandoning the whole process.

Once you've completed your log, spend time studying it to look for any patterns. Do this mindfully. Quiet your thoughts—especially your self-judgmental thoughts—and take time to be curiously attentive to what is happening when you go through this experience of putting food and drink into your body. Are you eating more, or more often, at certain times of day? Do certain feelings or body states trigger your reach for food? What prompts you to eat certain kinds of foods? What makes for a satisfying eating experience for you? What makes for a lousy eating experience?

Just by observing your behavior for three days, you may soon start to notice you're making changes in how, what, and when you eat. You're becoming *aware*. Use your journal, a drawing pad, a collage arrangement, or another creative venue to reflect further on what you're discovering about your relationship to food. You might find yourself eager to change your eating habits, even drastically, ready to map out a whole new plan related to nutrition, dieting, and so on. While I don't want to discourage such planning, I'm not recommending it. Too often, I've seen women (myself included) commit to making big changes in their eating—and then they don't follow through for more than a few days and end up feeling like failures. Instead, continuing to develop conscious awareness of your body and your eating practices will help to generate sustainable changes that flow more naturally from an inner-directed knowing.

While the Food and Feeling diary and the other exercises suggested in this chapter can support change by deepening your awareness of your food habits, some eating patterns and attitudes are so self-destructive that professional help is needed. Does looking at your Food and Feeling diary seem way too overwhelming or discouraging? Are you deliberately throwing up after you eat? Are you restricting your eating to the point that you're having negative health effects? If you feel totally out of control concerning your eating, please seek the help of a professional who is experienced in working with eating disorders.

EXERCISE: FOOD SAVORING

This exercise has been used in many settings to help people become more mindful about the process of eating. It's a reminder of the ecstasy that's possible from each bite of food when we are in a present-moment state of awareness.

Take one raisin (or a grape, an apple slice, or any tiny food item). Set it on a plate before you as if it were a banquet. Observe it with your eyes for a few minutes, noticing its color, shape, and all the variations of its surface. Bring it up to your nose and spend a few minutes savoring its aroma. Then put it in your mouth and take a long, long time to chew it before swallowing it. Chew it sixty times or more. Notice the feel of its texture and shape. Let its flavor linger on your tongue. Sit for a few minutes enjoying the completion of the experience before going on with your day.

What do you really want and need?

The above exercises are great warm-ups for developing an ongoing practice of conscious body awareness related to food. The Food and Feeling diary gives you an overview of your eating behavior patterns. This food-savoring exercise demonstrates the ideal of what ecstatic, present-moment eating can feel like. Now begins the ongoing work of moving inside the daily eating behavior patterns for a more concentrated process of awareness, redirection, and healing. What better way to start than with attention to what your body is trying to tell you?

At least once each day, when you feel like going for some food, stop and take a deep breath. Then take another one. Set aside whatever you're doing, delay briefly going for the food, and be still. Create an intention to listen with love to your body. Then do a body survey. As you did in the Food and Feeling diary, observe your body state but do so in more of a slow-motion fashion. What specifically is pulling you toward eating? Check your senses first. Is there a whiff of a pleasant aroma or a view of a tasty item within range? Now scan your entire body from foot to skull. Is there anything in your body that hurts? That feels "off"? Is there tension, pain, or strain anywhere? A backache? A nervous stomach? Pay particular attention to any discomfort in your stomach. Is it hunger? Or is it something else? *Maybe it's even a feeling of being stuffed.*

In my own tendency to food addiction, I've been driven to eat at times because of the discomfort I've felt from recently eating too much. The fuzzy logic of addiction spins me into denial of how full I am. Rushing to resolve the matter quickly, I become driven to cover over the uncomfortable feeling I'm having with something pleasurable, and food is the easiest solution (as well as my habitual "drug").

So take it slow with your body survey. Honestly give yourself enough time to check in with your body to notice whether food is really going to solve whatever stress or discomfort may be present. Even if it's only a pleasant aroma calling you to eat, being mindfully present in your body will help you determine whether eating at this time is appropriate for your health and well-being or whether simply enjoying the aroma makes more sense.

Face up to the hidden stress

Denise, while writing a complicated report for a client on her computer, has the thought, *I think I'll eat one of those apples I got yesterday.* She is momentarily aware that she just ate a short while earlier, but rationalizes that *it's healthy food and these apples are small. I'll just eat one.* Denise is learning to practice body awareness instead of eating every time she's uncomfortable, so she decides this is a good time to try it out.

Denise turns her attention to doing a body survey and quickly discovers that she's sitting a little cockeyed, her middle section leaning to the right and her shoulders to the left. She adjusts her position and notices that her breath automatically deepens when she's sitting upright. She takes two more conscious breaths, breathing even deeper. As she does, she's aware that her eyebrows are pulled together and her forehead feels scrunched up, with just a hint of a headache coming on. Her jaw is also clenched. *What's all this tension about?* she wonders. She decides to "listen" very closely to find out.

Denise doesn't try to relax or make any changes at all, even though she feels the tension in her face increase now that she has noticed these sensations. She wants to tune in to this messenger and learn from it. She gives her full, curious, and caring attention to her facial distress for a few minutes *without trying to change it,* but she observes any changes that do take place. As she becomes more familiar with what is happening in her face, she sincerely, compassionately asks, *What do you need right now?* This question is addressed to her face, the messenger for her distress. But it is more of an offer of help to her whole body, to her whole self: *How can I bring you relief?*

The thought of those apples in the refrigerator again comes to her mind. But Denise has become more present in her body now, and the pull to eat has weakened. Listening to her body has taken her deeper inside herself. Her mind is getting quieter, her body more relaxed. Denise had been working very hard on the report, and her mind had been straining to pull together the information in the right way. Now that she's maintained a period of attention to her body, she notices her senses are opening up. She hears the sound of the birds outside and the hum of the refrigerator. The words "lighten up" pop into her mind. She looks out the window, where a cardinal is poised on a branch, its feathers a bright red in the morning sun. She stands up, takes a deep breath, goes over to the window, and watches the cardinal for a while.

She turns her attention to her face and her whole self again, asking, *How can I bring you relief?* Her eyebrows suddenly rise and her cheeks widen, and what pops into her mind is, *Maybe I could lighten up on this project. I've gotten so narrowed in on it, pressuring myself to get every detail perfect, no wonder my face got scrunched up.* A small smile appears on Denise's face. *Yup, I'm going to lighten up a little. It's just a report, but I've been working on it like my life depended on it. Time to take the pressure off myself. Besides, I do better work when I'm relaxed. In fact, let me re-create my intention for the day to be of service in a loving and centered way.* Her smile widens, and she takes another deep breath. Her jaw loosens. She uses her hands to pat her cheeks, her jaw, her forehead, her eyebrows. She is giving her face a thank-you massage.

Denise returns to her work refreshed, without eating the apple. She did not need food; she needed a break and an attitude shift. By following her body's lead, she brought her attention firmly into the present moment. She gave herself a mental and physical break from her work (including an eye break from the computer), and she opened herself up to a holistic response that addressed the needs of her body, mind, and spirit. In the past, Denise had mostly ignored her body's clues except to think of them as a vague kind of discomfort, which she thought food might at least hide if not relieve. Now she is learning to listen more closely.

Listening to your body takes time, and it's subtle business. Denise may sometimes receive several body signals, representing a number of different stressors. To sort out what would be most helpful to her in any given moment, she needs to stay attentive to *one* of her body's signals for a long enough period of time to get to what's behind it. As she stays with the process of mindful attention, her body will either release the distress on its own (by prompting a shift in posture, for example), or she'll become aware of underlying mental and emotional disconnects so she can address them appropriately. Addressing these disconnects will be easier once she's in this body-centered, present-moment state of awareness. If more than one signal calls for her attention, she can use the same process for each one. Many times, once the most urgent issue is addressed, the resulting shift in body state and mental outlook has positive spinoff effects on other stressors.

The Breathe and Break exercise can be used with any kind of addictive tendency. The craving for any kind of "fix" is not about the desired *something* itself. It *is* an attempt to get you to fix or take care of something though, and your body is eager to give you clues about what that is. Some addictive substances, such as alcohol and illegal or certain prescription drugs, create biochemical changes in some people that make reading your body's signals more difficult. So do the effects of some health conditions and their medications. Nonetheless, your body will make heroic efforts to communicate an appropriate call for help when you experience physical, mental, or emotional discord. Before reaching for the usual false fix, let your body tell you what you truly need. It's the kind thing to do.

Get support

If your addiction is greatly disrupting your life, seek professional help. Also, dozens of Twelve Step groups, ranging from Overeaters Anonymous to Narcotics Anonymous to Co-Dependents Anonymous, are available in many communities. They provide a free, nurturing support system for overcoming your addiction.

What Does Your Body Have to Say?

OBSERVE AND REFLECT

ANGER INVENTORY: One clue to our addictions is what makes us angry or irritable. When we're upset, it's because we're not getting something we want. Each time you're angry over the next few days, pay attention to what's in the back of your mind. Is there something you're craving that you're not getting at the moment? Approval? Control? A chance to gamble? Sweets? Drugs? Getting to your TV or computer or work? Be honest. What is it that's nonessential yet is on your mind a lot and leaves you feeling frenzied when you can't get it? What does this craving or addiction cost you?

WRITE

REFLECTIVE JOURNALING: Journal on the above observations.

IRRATIONAL CRAVINGS: Write a few paragraphs, beginning with "When I pursue _____ [what I irrationally crave] in excess, what I really want is _____."

LIVE

BREATHE AND BREAK EXERCISE: Do the Breathe and Break exercise whenever you feel the urge to "use" something or someone in a desperate or illogical way to make you feel better or "escape." Here are the steps:

1. Delay the act of using for at least five minutes.

2. Still yourself and breathe deeply a few times.

3. Bring your attention to your body and do a survey of your sensations. What hurts or what feels uncomfortable, perhaps straining or creating pressure? What feels pleasurable? Do not attempt to

change any of this unless something simple, such as shifting your posture, will bring obvious relief.

4. Identify one area of body distress that seems most prominent or promising for this exercise.

5. Keep your attention on this area for an extended period of time, five to fifteen minutes or more. As you observe, settle deeply into your body and become still. Observe with interest and without judgment or expectation. Just be curious and caring toward this area of your body. Notice any changes that take place. If any thought of your "fix" comes to mind, give it a moment's glance but return your attention to your body and the stillness. If you have trouble keeping your attention on your body, give a running description aloud of what you notice: "My left shoulder is dropping a little. So is my right shoulder, but not as much. Just now, as it moved, I took a deep breath."

6. As gently and compassionately as possible, ask what this area needs and what you can do to help. Open yourself up to guidance from your mind, body, and spirit. Wait patiently for any changes you notice in the special body area, any images or sounds that enter your mind, any "knowing" that comes to you from your inner spirit, and any sensations or urges elsewhere in your body that might help you grasp what is needed. Take your time to tune in to these responses. Your wise inner self will show you what you need.

7. Let the responses guide you to some type of self-loving action that will bring relief. The relief may be physical and it may not. Some types of chronic or acute pain, for example, may not go away. But a spiritual insight about them or a fresh mental decision may bring a type of relief that will reduce or eliminate your craving for the false fix.

8. Show your body you appreciate it in some way for alerting you to what needed your attention, for serving as a guide to relief, and for keeping you from giving your life and your will away.

· · · · · · · · · · · · · · **Part 3** · · · · · · · · · · · · ·

Create with Abandon

*"We are makers, mothers, fabricators, poets. Even if our cre-
ation does not endure, our need to create it is eternal. This
passion to create defines our humanity. It explains why we
resonate with a creator-godhead. We share the urgency to
replicate ourselves, to make creatures and name them, to set
them in the midst of predicaments and tell their stories."*

—ERICA JONG, *What Do Women Want?*

· ·

CHAPTER 8

Let's Play

One fiercely hot summer day, I came home to find four little girls in bright-colored swimming suits lying on their bellies on my neighbor's blacktop driveway. Water was streaming down the driveway toward them from a hose held by a small boy. The children were giggling and squealing as the cooling water flowed around, under, and over them. They rolled around in the water, splashed and tumbled over each other, and argued to get turns holding the hose. Gauging by the volume of their laughter, their delight was ecstatic. As I walked by them to get my mail from the mailbox, it was all I could do not to throw myself down alongside them on the blacktop and join in the fun. I wanted to play, too!

What stopped me, I wonder? When was the point in my life at which rollicking on the ground like that became taboo, when being grown up meant containing myself and not looking foolish? Maybe you've wondered that yourself at times, when you've seen children playing freely without inhibition.

Have your lost your playfulness?

When I was a child, I often rolled down a hill in our farmyard. I would lie down, push off, and let gravity take charge—flipping and flopping my body over and over, flinging me at dizzying speed. But one day when I was halfway down, cramping stopped the fun and I noticed my first flow of blood. My entrance into womanhood meant an end to the free romping of childhood. My mission now was to master high heels, girdles, and proper restraint. No more hill-rolling allowed.

This was not the first or only type of play that came to a halt as I moved through childhood. The natural physical exuberance of children is systematically reigned in, starting when we're quite young. "We're taught early on to stop sensing the world," Joan Erikson is quoted as saying in *A Walk on the Beach* (by Joan Anderson), bemoaning the gradual shutdown of this playful adventurousness. Erikson, who along with her husband Erik is known for developing the theory of our identity processing through eight life cycles, told Anderson, "Parents say no to their toddlers all the time, when all their child wants to do is to sense the world around him. Pity, isn't it!"

From the perspective of her crone wisdom in her nineties, Erikson offered this antidote to our sensory shutdown: "Overdose on the senses is what I say, all the way through life." Her words reflect how she lived. The themes of sensuality and playfulness permeated her life and are evident in the counsel she offers in her exchanges with the book's author, Joan Anderson, a woman in her fifties at the time. "We all need to unlearn the rules that are set up for us by others," she told Anderson. Near the end of her life, Erikson became even more adamant about passing on her commitment to living with abandon: "Make time to play each day . . . We're asses if we don't."

How much is play a part of your life? How often do you romp with the freedom of a child?

For many women, their playful nature has become so tamped down that it can only come out when prompted by a few glasses of wine or in sexual activity. For the most part, propriety, respectability, fear, and self-consciousness reign. These women seem to be living out some version of the mantras that my mother imprinted into my mind and body when I was growing up: "Don't be silly!" or "What will people think?" No wonder addiction to approval is rampant. What prison walls these restrictive notions dropped into place around us!

Play for the fun of it

It's not that women don't play at all. Plenty of women take tennis rackets or golf clubs in hand regularly, or play cards or other table games. These and similar organized, competitive activities can be a lot of fun, and silliness does take over occasionally. But where is the freeform play that is creative and exploratory, physical and sensual? As Erikson said, "Look, there isn't anything that I do that I don't enjoy. If I do it then I enjoy it. But playful activities are the best because they are goalless, the result is unknown, and they are full of fantasy, imagination, and random discovery. What can beat that?"

I'm always on the lookout for women who exhibit a physically playful spirit. I must admit I was surprised to find a role model in Eleanor Roosevelt, who often comes off in film footage as stilted and stuffy in her appearance. When watching a public television documentary about her life, however, I was delighted to see scenes of her frolicking with her friends. They were rolling around on the ground, splashing in the water, climbing onto tree branches, chasing and even tickling each other, laughing raucously. I was also reminded of a scene in *A Walk on the Beach* in which Erikson invites her younger friend to go out on a boat ride with her, and the two of them giddily splash each other with water.

"Play is freedom," says psychotherapist and Adlerian educator Thomas Wright in an unpublished essay he shared with me. "Play is an altered state of consciousness, a 'time out' from ordinary activity, an intermezzo in the flux of daily life." It enables us to "rest, get perspective, collect our thoughts, follow our bliss, create, laugh, revive our spirits, listen to our muse, explore transcendence, and create meaning for our lives."

It is with that spirit in mind that I give out an assignment in my Writing Your Own Permission Slip class: find a new way to play this week and write about it. Class members have come up with both tame and playful stretches in their capacity to play. One woman gleefully designed an elaborate, comical treasure hunt in a public sculpture garden as a birthday present for a friend. Another reported experimenting with ways to get her big toe to her mouth as she had done as a baby. Other new play adventures that class members have undertaken include make-believe activities with grandchildren, writing funny poems, and inventing a new game with computer floppy disks.

Since I always do the same assignments as the class members, and I've taught the class many times, I've had to come up with many new ways to play. In one case—and I was in my mid-fifties then—I revisited an old way to play, one I had wanted to return to ever since I was sixteen. I decided to roll down a hill. I devoted most of chapter 3 in *Body Odyssey* to this story, and it is one of the stories readers of that book tell me they like the most. I think it bears repeating here.

From the time I turned fifty and my bleeding stopped, I kept my eye open for . . . a good-sized hill slanted just right and padded with thick grass. [Occasionally, I'd see one and feel] the longing to roll there, but I always passed on by. A foolish thing, I thought. People would see me. I'm not dressed for it. Another time.

I remembered a perfect hill one day, one I'd often passed. I smiled and felt a whoosh of adrenaline as I imagined reliving the long-ago thrill of free rolling, but I couldn't quite imagine going to this hill at my age and actually doing what I dreamed. Besides, the hill was near a walking trail and lots of dogs are let loose to romp there. Still, I wanted to roll once more. Maybe there's another hill like this, I started to imagine, one secluded enough for a private tumble, but I soon dismissed the thought. Such silliness, I heard my mother's voice echo through me.

One evening I went off on a bike ride with the idea of wanting to find a fresh way to play. (I had given that assignment to a class I was teaching, and I always do the assignments myself.) I veered off my usual route onto a short side trail that I knew dead-ended in a small woody area. As I rode along, I glanced to one side and saw a very narrow and steep hill, one that appeared to have been deliberately built from piled-up loads of dirt as if intended for dirt bike runs or winter sledding. I remembered seeing it the last time I'd been this way, but it newly caught my eye. Its fairly even surface, covered in grass, beckoned now as an ideal spot for rolling.

But I hadn't planned to roll, not tonight. I'd look foolish if anyone saw me. Again, such silliness. Still, this was an out-of-the-way place with little chance of anyone spotting me. Unable to convince myself, I passed on by, biking on to a little-used ballpark around the back side of the hill—an even more remote location. Maybe I could do my rolling on this side of the hill, I thought for a moment, but I quickly rationalized that it was too secluded if I got hurt while rolling.

I made a U-turn to head back, thinking, well, maybe yes, I would actually go for it. Yes, I'd roll down the front side of the hill before heading home. This would be my "new" way to play—at least a way I'd never played as a grown-up. Heading back around the hill, ready for my adventure, I was wearing a silly grin and feeling nervous.

Darn! Three kids were circling around on bikes near the bottom of the hill. Well, what if I invited them to roll with me? For a moment, I actually entertained that idea, but soon dismissed it as only a storybook notion, then watched as they quickly biked out of sight.

Now's my chance. Here's the hill I've wanted. Why wait?

I parked my bike and mounted the hill quickly. After taking one more look around to make sure no one was in sight, I lay on my side and started to roll—cautiously. After a few turns, I stopped. Can I really do this? Yes. I must. Go! Another half dozen spins and I could tell I was headed not down the hill but at an angle, rolling off to one side. Stopping again, I repositioned myself, pushed off, and rolled unhindered, body flipping and flopping fast, head spinning, stomach spinning, eyes sighting sky, grass, sky, grass, sky. Omigod, what if there are sharp rocks or big bumps? I tried to look up to check but instantly felt the added strain on my neck from rolling in this cockeyed position. I succumbed at last to the spinning, safe or not, and I rolled on and on and on all the way to the bottom—out of control.

No mother voice was stopping me now. There were no social mores to follow, no one to please or impress. It wasn't dignified. It wasn't pretty. But it was me—giving myself over to my own momentum, helped along by the forces of mother earth, giving in to freedom. I felt like Sam Keen, the trapeze novice at age sixty-one, who, when he couldn't seem to bring himself through a successful leap to the next swing one day, decided instead that it was a good day to practice falling. The only measure of success was the willingness to let go and enjoy the descent.

Sprawled at the bottom of the hill, I was relieved to find I was still breathing—and felt no big pain. The ground beneath me felt firm and stable. The sky was still swirling past me rapidly, so I closed my eyes. I felt a little nauseous and was suddenly achy in many places. Two or three minutes passed before I made my way to standing. On unsteady feet, I wobbled toward my bike.

After checking to see if each body part still worked as usual, I mounted the bike in slow motion. As I pressed on the pedal, a slight pain pinged momentarily through my right foot. My left knee felt slightly out of joint, so I shook it a little. There! It was all right.

Assured that I was safe and barely damaged, I smiled to myself and took a deep breath. I briefly looked back at the hill I had just conquered, not by arduous climbing to achieve some feat of endurance, but by letting myself surrender. I wished for a moment that someone had been there to watch, to say, "Good for you" or to laugh with me at my cautions and clumsiness. Then I wondered if anyone would think I was silly or crazy if I told them what I'd done. But I quickly dismissed these outdated concerns. What does it matter? I had simply done what I had longed to do for a very long time. I had rolled down a big hill, just like when I was a kid. Such silliness, indeed! Such fun!

Your body remembers how to play

What is an "old way to play" you'd like to revisit? What fun things have you stopped doing because they're "too silly" or "too childish" or for any other reason that suppresses your spirit?

A surprising number of women have told me they never played as a child or don't know how to play. In fact, even the class assignment to find a new way to play is one that many women tell me they find hard to accomplish. They want to play, but who's got time? Besides, they say, *what would I do if were going to play?*

We all played as children. If you grew up in an abusive, alcoholic, or otherwise restrictive or intimidating home environment, you may have had very little chance to play. But children always find some way to imagine, make-believe, and explore their world creatively. Even children in World War II concentration camps retained a priceless window to freedom through playful discoveries and imaginings, which they recorded on tiny scraps of paper that were found after the war.

How, then, can you revive your own freewheeling sense of play and wonder?

Even if playing seems an absent or distant memory to you, your body will remember if given a little prompt. Haven't you ever smelled cinnamon or lilac blossoms or some other familiar, pleasing aroma from childhood and immediately felt as if you were back in the long-ago place where that aroma gave you such pleasure? Look through the list below to identify any of the experiences that once brought you childhood delight. Go through the list slowly, with attention to your body as you retrieve and reactivate the cellular memory of the sights, sounds, smells, taste, and touch of these activities.

Paper dolls
Hide-and-seek
Playing house
Hiding under a blanket with a flashlight
Flashlight shadows on the wall
Watching clouds, looking for familiar shapes
Playing tag
Making sand sculptures
Wearing plastic lips
Pretending to be a movie star
Red Rover, Red Rover
Playing circus
Etch A Sketch®
Playing dress-up
Climbing a tree
Rolling in a pile of leaves
Blindfold games
Playing school
"Button, button, who's got the button?"
Jump-rope rhymes

What memories did the activities on this list bring up? What did you feel in your body as you recalled your experiences?

Chances are that you have no desire to revive some of these childhood activities at this time in your life, but others may be fun to try again. One evening my friends and I pulled out flashlights to create shadows on the wall as we had done as children, and we found that making outrageous shadows with our hands was still great fun in our fifties and sixties. Playing in the sand at the beach can be as delightful in adulthood as in childhood. In fact, in my community a major event every summer is the creation of huge sand sculptures by adults on a lakefront beach.

I think God gave some women grandchildren mainly so they could rediscover or learn new ways to play themselves. A woman named Gippy commented on my blog about this topic:

"Coming from a very abused and dysfunctional family, I am now living my childhood with my six-month-old, three-year-old, and thirteen-year-old grandsons. My thirteen-year-old actually taught me, from his birth on, how to play and have fun. We have had a fabulous time together— making mud pies, learning to swim, building snowmen and having snowball fights, going down slides and climbing monkey bars (well, that was a few years ago), and now learning computer programs together (he's the teacher!) I play cars and water games with my three-year-old and dance with my six-month-old. I believe they think their grandmom is silly, funny and full of laughter even with illness along the way."

Which childhood activity could be fun for you to try again, perhaps in a new form? How about using your "pretend" skills to create a skit for a charity fundraiser? For your next birthday, why not invite your friends to show up dressed like a famous person from your teen era? Watching clouds and imagining characters and creatures in the shapes you see never grows old.

EXERCISE: HOUSEHOLD OBJECTS REIMAGINED

More important than retrieving or reworking old play methods is finding a form of play that stimulates your imagination, fosters a sense of freedom and adventure, and gives you fresh ideas and energy. In one session of the Permission Slip class, I lay out in front of the group household objects such as a wire whisk from the kitchen, pliers, or scissors. I pass one object around the circle at a time, and each person mimes some creative use for the object, as a child might do in imaginative play. So the wire whisk is transformed into a hot air balloon, an "idea" above someone's head, an earring, a turkey baster, and dozens of other items, depending on how many times it gets passed around the circle.

Try this Household Objects Reimagined activity with a group of friends the next time you get together. It's fun to do as a party game. Warning: this activity leads to explosive laughter, and it's a great imagination stretcher. It can also be used to help a group member who is "stuck" concerning a problem she's facing. Once everyone's imagination gets triggered while playing with the objects, you can then pass the person's problem around the circle and continue the playfulness by having each person imagine the problem in a fresh way. A group member's lazy co-worker, for example, might be seen as a sluggish tortoise, an unpaid holiday, or a train going nowhere. The goofier, the better. Seeing the problem playfully from a number of new perspectives can help stimulate fresh approaches to solving it.

Once, when I was teaching the Permission Slip class and I gave the "new way to play" assignment, I was in a sour frame of mind. I had no desire to play at all, let alone find a new way to play. I made plans to meet with a friend, Cynthia Ryden, who was taking the class, so we could jointly create a new way to play. When I got to her home for our play date, I told her I was depressed, and she said that she, too, was feeling down.

We talked for a while about how, when we're depressed, we don't easily want to give up being depressed. It probably has something to do with low serotonin levels creating inertia. We decided the only way we were willing to play was to poke fun at ourselves for hanging on to our depression. Before long we were writing a poem about it, and pretty soon we were giggling at our own "angst." Then we put the words to music and sang at the top of our lungs to a lilting melody. We even added a little marching step in time to the music and made frowning faces on paper plates to carry as banners while we sang, as if we were in a parade. We laughed like giggly teens and, needless to say, our depression took a walk. I can't sing the song for you on these pages, but use your imagination as you read the lyrics:

How I Love My Depression

It is noble, it is right
To be depressed with all our might
It's a perfect way to fight off
Good news and life's delight

We never will cheer up
We have to drink a cup
Of grimness, darkness, and hard luck

We love our somber state
With too much on our plate

How we love our depression (*twice*)

No matter how bright the day
We will never be sunny and gay
It's against our religion

We're proud of our plight
Happiness is a blight
We've climbed the height of depression

Don't talk of endorphins
We'd rather be orphans
Lonely and down in the dumps

Don't try to cheer us
We like to fume and fuss
We'd rather take our lumps

How we love our depression (*twice*)

Join in our misery
Wallow in self-pity
Linger in unhappiness all day long

It's not hard to belong
Just join in our song

How we love our depression (*twice*)

© 2001, Cynthia Ryden Austin and Pat Samples

Play and pray

Playing is also a spiritual exercise. It's a present-moment experience. When fully engaged in play, you lose any sense of time. There is only *now.* Your body feels vibrantly alive. Aches and pains fade from awareness. Laughter often erupts, and life seems lighter. Spiritual masters are often described as childlike. They delight in simple things, and most everything seems to them like play—which is a good reminder that play does not have to be a big, expensive, or time-consuming activity. Watching a butterfly, observing the patterns of bubbles in your dishwater, or singing a silly song can lighten your spirit and produce an experience of transcendent oneness with all that is.

What Does Your Body Have to Say?

OBSERVE AND REFLECT

PLAYTIME RERUN: Pull out of storage favorite items from childhood, photos, or other memorabilia that will help you remember how you used to play. Listen to recordings of children's songs such as "London Bridge" or "Old MacDonald Had a Farm." Go to an antique or thrift store and look for Tinkertoys or other toys familiar from childhood. Do whatever it takes to revive memories and physical feelings from the fun times in your early life. Select one activity that feels good in your body as you recall it—and do it again. Notice how you feel as you do it now. Notice any resistance or taboo thought that comes up, such as "This is silly" or "I'm too old for this." Whose opinion or *voice* is that? How does this taboo feeling affect your ability to enjoy what you enjoy?

NONSENSE CHANT: Recall some nonsensical saying or chant from childhood such as "If you step on a crack, you'll break your mother's back." Repeat the saying over and over, using the inflections you did as a child. Close your eyes as you continue saying it, and let any related sounds, sights, smells, activities, and feelings that are pleasurable come back to you. How could such nonsensical, but sensually satisfying, fun be a part of your life today?

WRITE

MAKE-BELIEVE WRITING: Write a few paragraphs, beginning with "When I was free to play and make-believe . . ."

LIVE

GOOD TIME PROBLEM-SOLVING: Being playful is always a good way to approach problem-solving. When you dread taking on some task or can't find your way out of a dilemma, ask yourself, "How can I have a good time doing this?" Consider singing or dancing your way through it, imagining it as something else (as in the Household Objects Reimagined exercise), or pretending it's a game.

CHAPTER 9

Move It, Shake It, Sing It, Stage It

W e're born to dance. I believe that's true from the center of my
bones. Something in us loves swirling and twirling, gliding and
dipping. We thrill to the freedom of our body moving through space. It's
a pleasantly dizzying and risky experience. Our whole self comes alive.

Move everything

I once watched a performance by a troupe of children from Uganda who
were dancing with unrestrained exuberance, using every muscle in their
bodies. Their hips and bellies were in constant motion, gyrating and shaking in ways I doubt my body has ever moved. As I watched, I wondered
what it would feel like to move *everything* like that. Surely, one could not
be depressed after such a dance.

The closest I come to this kind of full-body movement is whenever
I'm experiencing back strain or other body tensions and I decide to dance
myself loose. I can't dance standing up; that might hurt too much and
might even exaggerate the tension. So I lie down on the floor, listen to
some African dance music or other feverish rhythms, and start my body
shaking. At first I just shake my hands or feet, but after a while the music
entices my whole body to get into the act. Everything that can move *moves*.
Sometimes my movements became frenetic, as if I'm unleashing everything

I'm holding in. The experience is pleasurable and tension-relieving. Afterward, I feel full of energy.

Dancing of any type, whether done lying down or standing, not only relieves tension and stimulates the flow of energy—it's also a creative and satisfying means of self-expression. When done in the company of others, it leads to communication that goes beyond words. "Movement was our primary language when we were born," begins chapter 16 in my book *Body Odyssey.* "Then we learned words, and this native 'tongue' was mostly silenced. What if, as adults, we again embraced this elemental mode of communicating that came to us so naturally? If we created more occasions to romp and play together, wouldn't we be more connected and creative? If each of us trusted and enjoyed the movement and messages of our bodies, wouldn't we take better care of them—and communicate more honestly and vibrantly? If we danced together with those unlike us, could we even perhaps reduce the chance of going to war?"

Every week I lead a group of women in a movement improvisation session called Free Motion, which I described briefly in chapter 1 of this book. Sometimes we are upright as we move; sometimes we're on the floor. Our purpose is to let our inner impulses direct our dancing—to move as we are *moved.* In *Body Odyssey,* I describe what happens during a Free Motion session:

....

I may give some general direction—"Move lightly," "Let your movements be circular," "Move like you have nowhere to go"—but we each take great latitude in shaping that suggestion into a form. The "circular" movements may be someone's arms swinging around at her sides, or someone's whole body swirling in big swoops, or someone's feet rotating as she lies on her back.

Sooner or later, we always end up intersecting, moving in communication with one another. We bend, leap, and roll among each other, becoming, as one member put it, "bodies cooperating." The choreography is collaborative. Each of us creates forms from our internal impetus—the brushing, intertwining, and cradling of each other's heads, arms and hands, torsos, legs and feet. We can spend anywhere from a few minutes to an hour playing with a hundred ways of letting our hands be in conversation or folding ourselves over and around each other with childlike ease. We lose ourselves in getting to know the beauty and touch of our bodies in motion.

Sometimes we make faces, telling our stories with all forty-five muscles. We are giving witness to what theologian and philosopher Thomas Moore, in Care of the Soul, *says about the face being "a map of the soul." Drooped eyes, wrinkled brows, a wide grin, or sunken cheeks are markers of spirit. During our dance sessions, our faces have a chance to expand into full repertoire and reveal both well-marked and subtle terrains.*

How does your body move when it's free to move? What happens when you give your face a chance to dance? Or, like many women, do you think you "can't" dance or that it would be embarrassing to do anything so foolish, or that you can only dance on a public dance floor with a partner?

I once led a Body Odyssey retreat at an assisted living facility. In places like this, the body's limitations are often emphasized, and people sit unmoving much of the day. That day I invited the people living there to discover all the gifts their bodies have to offer. I asked them what their bodies had done in their lifetimes. Skating. Picking rocks. Dancing. Holding a grandchild. Sewing. Whistling. Shaking hands. Sewing.

All of our bodies have been busy. They carry in them a lot of stories. And many of these stories are still living stories. Even when someone sits in a wheelchair and parts of her body can't move, other parts—perhaps her hands, jaws, and eyelids—may be free to tell these stories. The people I was with that day found more of the "life" living in their bodies, the capabilities they still had. Before long, they were doing hand dancing, their bent and wrinkled limbs waving gracefully through the air. Some people took turns leading the dance, while the rest followed their movements. One woman, after the session, told me she found this dancing to be meditative. She said her thoughts were normally preoccupied with sadness about her estranged relationship with her son. During the dancing, all thoughts of her son and her sadness disappeared.

Another woman, who talked with excitement about her memories of dancing, said she had given up dancing after she had a stroke. She refused to join the rest of us in the simple dance form of moving our hands through the air.

How often, it seems, we get stuck in thinking something can only be done a certain way. If she couldn't dance on her feet, this woman thought it was impossible to dance. Watching her and feeling sad that she was missing out on the fun, I was reminded to stay open to new possibilities myself, to refuse to let my aliveness be limited even when challenges come my way.

We can always dance. In one of my Body Odyssey workshops, a man who is quadriplegic even found a way to dance, weaving his head and neck to the music. It was beautiful to behold. He hadn't given up on dancing. He knew what it meant to live!

Lift your spirits through the arts

Dancing, acting a theatre role, or singing—any form of artistic creation can lift our spirits and express what's inside us. "The arts give us tools to get at our essence," says Anthony Hyatt, a musician and the co-director of Quicksilver, a creative dance troupe based in Bethesda, Maryland, that is made up of women in their seventies and eighties. Most of the women in Quicksilver didn't begin to dance until late in life, and their primary goal is not excellence in performance (though their occasional onstage performances have been well received) but to bring out their creativity and express what's simmering inside themselves. They meet weekly for creative movement and sometimes performance rehearsals. Once a month, they accompany Hyatt to local senior centers and senior living campuses and serve as role models of creativity while inviting the people there to join with them in the dancing.

All across the country, older adults are finding ways to enjoy creative arts activities that contribute not only to their own well-being but to their community. Members of Kairos Dance Theatre in Minneapolis, led by artistic director Maria Genné, go twice a week to an adult day care center to involve the elders there in creative dance activities. Genné draws out their stories through movement and then choreographs those movement stories into full-blown professionally staged dance numbers. The elders all have health problems, some quite serious, yet many of them regularly participate onstage in the many public performances by the intergenerational company that includes members from preschool age to people in their eighties.

Pass on your legacy

In New York City, the Pearls of Wisdom is a multicultural group of elder storytellers who take their stories of struggle and strength, heartache and humor, into community venues. They incorporate dramatic techniques as they tell their stories and sometimes include music and dance. Pearls of Wisdom is part of a citywide, long-running program called Elders Share the Arts that creates opportunities for older adults to become involved in the arts. The group members are particularly interested in sharing their stories with children, to help pass along their cultural heritage and their zest for life. "Young people look through the windows of our memories and find assurances that life is worth living and striving for," Amatullah Saleem told the 2005 Mini-Conference on Creativity and Aging in America.

Senior theatres are another outlet for creative expression. About seven hundred senior theatres exist across the United States, giving people over fifty a chance to do what we all loved to do as kids—play-act. Most use prepared scripts, but others write their own scripts through scene development work under the guidance of theatre professionals. In Douglas County, a rural county in western Minnesota, Kathy Ray, a playwright and theatre director, visited with dozens of the area's older citizens to gather and record remembrances of their childhood days. She then worked with a small group of them to shape these stories into a theatre revue, first introducing them to basic theatre staging and playwriting skills to get them started. The revue was staged in a public community production that included an intergenerational cast—and some of the playwrights. For many of the performers, it was their first appearance in a play. For the playwrights, performers, and the community, the whole adventure was a process of discovery, celebration, and community-building.

One of the Douglas County performers, Marjorie Van Gorp, age eighty-two, donned a man's suit a couple sizes too large for her and whittled with a jackknife as she portrayed her father on stage. In the (imagined) words of her father, Van Gorp told of his emigration from Sweden to America as a young man with his mother after his mother's grandfather and brother were killed in a railroad accident while working to get money to buy their own land here. "It was quite an emotional experience," Van Gorp told me. "It seems that, after writing all this and playing my father, I felt a little closer to him. I could never tell his story without having my voice crack."

Try on new roles

The performing arts offer wonderful opportunities to play roles that reflect different aspects of our character and learn more about ourselves and our world. They provide a venue to discover and express our emotions. We also get a chance to try on unfamiliar roles, giving us experience in fresh ways of behaving. In addition, playing someone else can help us to understand better how other people feel and think. Through imaginative portrayals, we're able to try on with our whole being new ways of thinking and being.

A few years ago, I saw a notice in my local paper for a play audition. I thought it would be fun to try out. I had been feeling a little "flat" and wanted something to perk me up. To my surprise, I got cast as the queen mother—a pompous, overbearing character prone to issuing orders. I took on the role with trepidation, having only acted onstage a few times when I was quite young. But it turned out to be the perfect part for me.

First of all, playing this character demanded lots of energy and volume. Since I spend much of my everyday life quietly writing at my desk, the experience gave me the perk-up I desired.

Even more significant was how much I learned from playing this all-too-familiar character. Coming from a family with a domineering mother, I grew up developing a bossy bent myself. This need to be in control has, at times, alienated people around me, made it difficult for me to work for a boss, and generated anxiety when things don't go my way. While I have worked with some success to change this tendency through therapy and other means, it still drives my bus more than I'd like. Out of shame, I often try to hide or suppress this unpleasant aspect of my character. Of course, what gets hidden becomes a menacing "shadow" that pops up unexpectedly in moments of stress, further adding to my shame.

The queen mother role gave full stage to my shadow. Rather than hide my bossy tendency, I got to feel it fully and even flaunt it. Prancing around the stage, I could freely make demands and order people around. I felt foolish but, at the same time, I enjoyed playing this part. Here was a safe, creative forum for my suppressed feelings. I could play them out without hurting anyone. In fact, I was entertaining people and making them laugh.

Playing this role also made *me* laugh—at myself. By acting out my controlling tendencies in such an exaggerated manner, I could more easily sense their absurdity. I also became more conscious of how this way of behaving was a character role I had assumed early in life. It was an "act" that wasn't the real me. And just as I could stop playing the queen mother after the show, I had the possibility of shedding this way of thinking and behaving in my everyday life.

I wish I could say I've never been bossy or demanding since. Not so. But I now more easily recognize my "queen mother" character when it shows up, and I feel less driven by it. Occasionally, in the privacy of my own living room, I even assume an arrogant queen mother pose and spout a few pompous lines until the feeling passes.

What is your performance fantasy? What stories would you like to tell? What roles would you like to act out? *But,* you might protest, *I'm no actress.* Yes, you are. As a child, you made up stories and characters all the time. Even if grown-ups scoffed at your "nonsense," you didn't quit performing completely. Think about it. Haven't you "acted" out a few dramatic scenes in your adult life? Consider your fine performances of righteous innocence when you've made a mistake that you're sure won't be found out. What about the times you so enthusiastically said, "I'll call you" when you didn't really mean it? Or when you pretended to know something you didn't?

We all "perform" at times, usually to avoid trouble or in hopes of getting love and approval. But what if you tapped into that same creative potential to express yourself artistically—alone in your own living room, with a community of friends, or onstage before an audience? You don't have to be a pro or even call yourself an artist, but you can explore dance, acting, singing, or other art forms as a way to give your body a pleasurable venue for self-discovery, self-expression, and contribution to the community.

It's good for you

If these benefits aren't enough to persuade you to get going, consider this: the arts are good for your health. A landmark study of creativity and aging by George Washington University scholar Gene Cohen, MD, PhD, shows that older adults who participate in professionally led arts programs demonstrate marked health benefits, including not only lower depression rates and less loneliness, but fewer medications, falls, and doctor visits than those who don't take part. If you want to improve your chances of living a long and satisfying life, treat yourself to the fun and freedom of participation in the arts. Your body will thank you.

Join in the fun

Here are a few ways you can get connected with performing arts activities in your community:

- Get involved in a community theatre.
- Check out your local high school or college theatre to see if they could use an adult to play a role in one of their productions.
- Create or participate in a performance group within your faith or cultural community (e.g., a choir, pageant, sacred dance).
- Rehearse and then make an audio or video recording of yourself telling an important story from your life. Share it with family and friends.
- Start or join a group that does informal dramatic play readings together.
- Join a community choir.
- Start a singing group just for fun.
- Meet regularly with a group of women friends in someone's family room or party room to do improvisational dancing together.
- Volunteer to read stories to children at schools and preschool programs, and read them with full dramatic flair.

- Take a theatre, dance, or singing class at a local studio or school.
- Start or join a drumming group or a band.
- Take music lessons.
- Go to a place that features karaoke—and sing!

What Does Your Body Have to Say?

OBSERVE AND REFLECT

CONFLICT PLAY-ACTING: When you're having a conflict with someone, play-act a scene by yourself that you two might have when arguing. Take on the other person's persona and point of view when it's that person's turn to talk in your imaginary dialogue. Try sincerely to step inside his or her way of being as if you were living inside that person's body and world. See if this experience gives you any insights that may help you in relating to that person in real life.

DRAMATIZING A STORY: In a group with other women, share stories about some particular theme such as lost loves, favorite jobs, or sacred moments. Work together to create a dramatic story from one of these stories or a mix of them. Identify the characters, the setting, the time (e.g., 1960s, morning), and specific actions and dialogue that will set the scene, show development of a conflict or tension, and create a turn of events that leads to resolution and a conclusion. Let one person serve as director. Have fun with this. Come up with makeshift props and some hint of costumes and set, but keep the trappings simple. Put your attention on developing the story so it makes sense and so that someone watching can follow and enjoy the drama that unfolds. Encourage and help each other. You can perform for friends and family, a local senior living campus, school, or other group if you wish. Or you can just enjoy among yourselves the satisfaction of creating the performance. Afterward, spend time sharing the discoveries you each made from this experience.

WRITE

DESCRIBE YOUR CHARACTER: Write a description of yourself as if you were writing out instructions for someone to play you as a character in a play. How would you say you look, walk, breathe, laugh? What is your vocal quality, your pattern of speech? Make up a scene and describe how you would be portrayed in that scene. Then, play-act that scene in a highly melodramatic way. What did you learn about yourself? Do the same for other significant people in your life, and see what you discover about them.

LIVE

DANCE ROUTINES: Dance your way through your morning dressing, bathing, and hair care routines. Dance around your kitchen as you prepare a meal.

SONGS TO GO: Make up songs about your life and sing them at the top of your lungs as you drive in your car.

GRANDCHILDREN PLAY-ALONG: Get on the floor with your grandchildren and act like animals or storybook characters.

CHAPTER 10

Making Full-Bodied Agreements

All day long we make agreements to do certain things. *Yes, I'll meet with you. Sure, I'll stay until you get back. Okay, I'll finish that report.* But even as we say yes, our body may signal that we're not in full agreement with what we're deciding or saying.

Let's say that you're most creative and productive in the early morning. When a good friend wants to meet you for breakfast—the only time she's available—you say yes, though you hate to get a late start on an important project that requires your sharpest thinking. While you're with your friend, you feel a nagging tension in your lower back. In fact, you're not fully attentive to what she's saying because of your back discomfort. You cut short your visit so you can get to a comfortable chair with good back support. The rest of the day you're taking pain pills and applying a heating pad off and on. You can hardly concentrate on your important project.

In this example, you're "of two minds," and your body is making sure you recognize the split. Much of our body distress arises from living in a state of *dis*agreement with what's going on around us, or among conflicting needs and desires within us. Paying attention to our physical state as we make decisions and say yes and no can help us enter with integrity into full-bodied agreements.

Get to know the feeling of yes and no

What does a full-bodied agreement feel like? Think back to a recent experience when you said an enthusiastic, unequivocal yes to someone. You were so clear about your intention and attention that you were there 100 percent—in the *now*. Recapture in your body that same experience now. Feel again the full engagement, the *yes*. Chances are you feel warmth in your body, a sense of vitality or energy flowing through you. Notice any other specific physical sensations associated with the experience. Notice what yes feels like.

How often do you live in this full-bodied state of yes? Few of us live there all the time. We often feel torn—wanting to do more than one thing at a time or wanting to escape something that is happening. Are there major areas of your life where you feel torn right now? Do you have mixed feelings about staying in your job or career? Are you in limbo about any of your relationships? What about moving away or staying where you live?

Even in your day-to-day decisions, you may experience ambivalence. Have you said yes or no to certain things halfheartedly today? Are you second-guessing some of your decisions? Are you still wavering about what to choose?

None of these states of mind are wrong. We're faced with hundreds of decisions each day, and some of them require a good bit of information gathering and reflection before making a choice. We read labels to determine the healthiest food to buy. We compare flight schedules and prices before buying a ticket. We weigh pros and cons before deciding to go to a concert with friends or accept a job offer. Yet at some point we decide—or at least declare we've decided. That decision or declaration can have many nuances.

Try this experiment. Stand up and practice saying yes in the various ways listed below, letting your voice and whole body vary accordingly. Say yes as if you're:

- Giving in
- Feeling shy about it
- Feeling defiant
- Doing it to manipulate someone

- Making fun of the asker
- Being brave
- Being playful
- Eager

Do the same process with no. Say no as if you're:

- Defiant
- Doubting yourself
- Carefree
- Angry
- Being playful
- Being flirtatious
- Being insulting

As you can tell from this experiment, *yes* and *no* are not simple words nor are they just mental activity. They're connected with emotions—and the more emotions associated with a decision, the more our body gets into the act. Often, in fact, our emotions run our decisions. We make or break an agreement based on how we feel at that moment. At times, our body, mind, and emotions all seem at odds as we enter into an agreement.

Let's say you're in a book club and the group is choosing the next book to discuss. You love reading women's books on personal empowerment, but two other group members are advocating for a best-selling political novel, an especially long one at that. A whole range of thoughts, feelings, and sensations show up for you: *These women are so smart about what's going on in the world; I'll feel very ignorant discussing current politics, though I don't really care that much about politics anyway. We read their choice last time; it's someone else's turn. I should have come prepared with something to suggest. With this hot flash and my arthritis pain going on right now, I'd better not speak up; I'll just sound cranky. Anyway, I just want to get this decision over with. What the heck, let them have their way.*

When the time comes for a vote, you say, "OK," but the internal dissonance in your mind may continue all the way home from the meeting, and nag at you every time you pick up the book to read. That dissonance is reflected in your body. You may squirm in your seat. Your forehead may wrinkle. A headache might surface. The lingering dissonance results from an incomplete decision. It's trying to reconcile yes, no, yes, no.

Practice the art of completion

To make a full-bodied agreement requires completion. In our high-speed, multitasking world, you may be like most people, rarely taking time to complete something fully before moving on to something else. As you hang up the phone with one hand, your other arm is slipping into your coat so you can rush out the door. Leftover thoughts, feelings, and sensations from your phone conversation continue in the background (sometimes in the foreground) as you get behind the wheel of your car and drive off. I suspect that many accidents, at home and on the road, result from this incomplete, distracted way of living. Making full-bodied agreements calls for completion. The "Yes, I'm finished with this conversation" is a separate act from "Yes, I'm leaving to go to my appointment." For each of these acts to be completed requires awareness, which can begin with the simple act of breathing.

Right now, you've just completed reading the previous paragraph. Say yes to that. Take a breath. Rest. In doing so, you're practicing present-moment awareness, which involves feeling complete with each experience you have. Each agreement, when it's made consciously and fully, is done. The act of breathing that follows, when done in a restful, conscious way, becomes its own complete experience. It's like the space between the period at the end of a sentence and the capital letter that begins the next one, or like the rest in a musical score.

That doesn't mean you won't revisit some decisions and make new choices. But once you make a conscious, full-bodied choice, in that moment you're no longer "of two minds." The decision is complete. Then you can rest, however briefly, until the next decision. Rest adds space into the agreement. It gives it room to live, as the soil provides room for a seed. This is no small matter. In this space of completion, of rest, of stillness, you are delivering your decision into the universe. You are giving your yes as an act of creation. The universe can't help but respond with its own yes in return, organizing its resources to support your choice.

Should I or shouldn't I?

For many women, making decisions is difficult. Why is that? In our early years, we learned that men were in office and in power, and making decisions was their rightful place. Besides, women weren't smart enough to make good choices. The "dumb blonde" jokes are passé now, but along with centuries of disregard for women's contributions, they've left their mark. As women, we're also supporters and nurturers by nature and by cultural assignment, so the decisions of others tend to take precedence over our own. "What do *you* think?" "No, you pick first." This drive to be supportive, along with a hunger to be accepted and included, frequently morphs into exaggerated people-pleasing and approval-seeking. "What will people think?" "Am I doing this right?" Deference and self-doubt can turn nearly every decision into a second-guessing exercise.

By midlife, many of us have become more self-assured. Some have gained broad experience in making big and tough decisions in various leadership roles. We're confident decision-makers much of the time. Yet lingering hesitations and doubts remain, long embodied from prior history. Plus, we're swamped by a growing deluge of decisions to make in our high-information world, with multitudes of consequences to consider. So much is at stake in our decisions. So much can go wrong.

Consult your body

Our body registers all these uncertainties and related fears. Simply put, we feel stress. Sometimes we feel so overwhelmed with all the decisions we face, our body goes into survival mode. We literally feel like curling up and hiding. We crave a return to the fetal position—to a safe, nurturing place where someone else handles all the decisions. Pain or illness may surface or increase in order to give us a good excuse for curling up in bed. Addictive habits may surface. We reach for alcohol, food, busyness, or other fixes for our relief. Our body is asking for relief all right, but any temporary fix won't satisfy the distress that comes from living in a state of dissonance and fear. Instead of masking the distress, we can turn to our body as our guide and resource.

A wise friend once told me that when she is faced with a difficult decision, she gives each option a day's test. She chooses one option and tries it on for twenty-four hours to see how it feels. She walks, talks, and thinks in ways that reflect that decision. Then she gives the same trial period to the opposite choice. I've found this method especially helpful when making major decisions such as whether to end a relationship or make a job shift.

You can try this same process. Bring to mind a decision you're facing, and use my friend's twenty-four-hour test to explore the yes and no more fully. Or you can spend a few minutes right now embodying each option by using one of the following exercises.

EXERCISE: IMAGINE YOUR DECISION COMPLETED

Write down your choices, so each one is clearly spelled out: (1) Yes, I will _____. (2) No, I won't _____. Settle back in your chair, quiet your mind, and relax your body. Say the first choice to yourself and then let your imagination play out as fully as you can what will happen once this choice is made. In particular, imagine and *feel* the sensory and energetic aspects of this choice. What sights or sounds are associated with it? What physical position and state of movement are you in? Notice your body temperature, your energy level, your level of ease or anxiety. Envision your interactions with others and again *sense* this experience as fully as you can.

As you observe your body state, be aware of any particular part of the body that asks for attention. Treat this body part as your friend and messenger. As you have learned to do in previous chapters, stay closely attentive to what is happening in this area of your body, and give it a "voice" in some way (through movement, words, sounds, and so on). Let it speak until you have learned what it is asking of you and you have attended to its needs. When you have done so, check with your body to see if any other area(s) also need attention, and follow the same process. Finally, observe your overall sense of well-being. Then write in your journal, starting with "By saying yes, I _____."

Now do the same process based on a "no" decision. When you're finished, you will be able to make your decision by drawing not only on external evidence but on your body wisdom as well.

EXERCISE: PLAY-ACT YOUR CHOICES

Have some fun with your decision-making process. Stage a dramatic debate or create a series of scenes representing your various choices. Do this by yourself, or invite a friend or support group to be your audience. Give each choice a full staging by giving an unrehearsed but passionate speech on behalf of each position. Or play out different characters involved in the choice. Or give each of the different "voices" within your mind a role. Get your whole body into the act, letting your voice express the emotions associated with a particular choice, gesturing and moving around to play out scenarios and using props. You may be surprised at the thoughts or feelings that bubble up as you allow yourself to go a little crazy on "stage."

You can set up this dramatic staging for yourself in several ways:

- Stage the scene as an interview. Pretend you're Oprah interviewing two characters, one representing each of your choices. Then step into each "character" and respond, using your whole body to give life to that point of view. If you're with a friend or group, have someone else play Oprah's part.

- Use a different setting for each choice. Sit in one chair to advocate for one choice, in another chair to advocate for the opposite choice. Or, use a different room to play out each option you're considering. If you're feeling as if your life will be "in the toilet" by making a particular choice, maybe you could stage a scene in the bathroom. If one choice feels like going on a long journey, stage it in a hallway. The more playfully and metaphorically you act out the choices, the more likely you'll get a fresh perspective on the situation. New, more satisfying options might even emerge.

- A little costuming can help you get into character. Put on a different hat or jacket or scarf for each position to establish the appropriate *attitude*.

- Try out saying each choice in different voices. Let's say you're deciding how to tell your boss you're quitting. Declare your resignation with a discouraged voice, a righteous voice, and an enthusiastic voice. As you physically feel into these voices and as you hear how they sound, you'll get a better sense of what feels like "home" and what kind of energy you'll be giving off. If friends are present for your staging, have someone play your boss.

After playing out these scenes, your decision will move from a mental exercise to a full-bodied experience. You'll feel the *energy* present in the various points of view. You'll have *more* energy—more aliveness— to bring to the decision. You'll find it easier to move off "stuck" and into action.

Once you've reached a decision, declare it aloud at full volume. Let the decision vibrate all the way to the core of your bones. Make the choice as if the decision matters, as if your opinion matters, as if *you* matter. Then, leave the other choice(s) behind, and take a breath. Your choice is complete. The universe can now line up behind you.

Say no with your whole body

In some of my workshops, I hand each person a small card with the word "no" on it. I say, "Some of you may not be familiar with this word," and the room erupts in laughter, especially when the audience is mostly women. Women have a hard time saying no. We're such givers. We've learned that our role is to help, to please, to make it easy for others.

Yet there are times we want to, and must, say no. I used to get involved in relationships with men who were quirky and gabby. I'd find them to be bright and interesting at first, but then they'd talk on and on and on, way beyond the point of my interest. I'd sit there and politely listen until I thought I'd go crazy. I couldn't bring myself to tell them I didn't want to listen anymore. I might hurt their feelings. They needed a friend. Blah, blah, blah. My whole body was screaming *no*, but there I sat, smiling and nodding with feigned interest. I was lying. I pretended to care about what they were saying when I didn't.

So I wasn't really being a good friend after all. I needed to say, *"No! Stop!"* Instead, I was saying no to myself. I was stopping myself. As a result, I'd endure headaches, neck tensions, and any number of other signals that I was living this lie. I heard my body speaking emphatically, but I'd ignore it or try to quiet it down. I hadn't learned how to listen to my body with love.

Now when I feel a *no* rippling through my nervous system, I listen. I may not be able to confidently and courageously *say* that no right away. Fears of hurting the other person or of saying the wrong thing still arise. That's not all bad. I truly do not want to be mean or make the other person wrong. Still, I want to say no. No, I'm not willing to listen to you anymore. No, I will not work any more hours on this project today. No, you cannot live in my house anymore without paying rent.

To have the clarity and confidence to say no, I call on my body for help. One way I do that is to recall an instance from my past when I was able to say no with full authority. I then recapture the state my body was in during that experience, readopting my physical stance, vocal qualities, movements, and other qualities from that experience.

The experience I usually recall is the moment I told my husband I would no longer stay in our marriage. A certain behavior of his showed up *once again*, and I'd had it. *No more!* I felt in every cell of my body the certainty and power of that decision. It actually helped that I was having PMS at the time. My hormonal impatience didn't allow any room for my usual deferent niceness or the wavering self-doubt that had kept me in the marriage way too long. I was fed up, done, and ready to move on, what-ever that would take. When I recall and re-embody the crisp firmness of my voice, the tall erectness of my torso, and the erupting energy spreading out to all my extremities, I can draw on the certainty and power I felt at that moment to say a full-bodied no in my current situation. Once my body takes the lead, my mind follows.

Try this yourself. Think of an experience when you declared a firm no, when you said it with everything in your body. Revisit the sensory and energetic memory of that moment. What was your pulse rate? Where did you feel heat in your body? How were you standing, speaking? What did your hands do? Revive those sensations, those feelings, with as much intensity as you can. Then bring your attention to a current situation in which you've been hesitating to say no, and bring that same energy to it. Feel into the no. Feel its certainty, its power. *Be* the no.

Exercise: Let Your Fist Say It First

In some of my workshops, I teach participants how to practice saying an authentic, full-bodied no. You can try this exercise yourself. Stand with your left foot two lengths ahead of your right one. Extend your left arm forward palm down and curl your hand into a fist. Place your right arm at your side, with the elbow pointed backward and your right hand palm up, curled into a fist. In slow motion, practice switching the position of your arms simultaneously. Your left arm comes back to your side, rotating so that the left fist is turned palm up. The right arm extends forward, with the fist turned palm down. Your back remains erect as you move forward. Do not lean or bend forward. Practice alternating your arm positions several times, slowly, until you can do it smoothly. Then, each time the right arm extends forward, add the movement of the right foot stepping forward on the floor so that your right knee is lined up under the elbow of the extended arm. When the right arm comes back, the right foot returns to its original position.

Once you can do these alternating movements smoothly, shift into super high speed when you move your right hand and foot forward. Bring your right arm forward as a sharp thrust, quickly, as if you were trying to punch a hole in the wall. Once you can do this swiftly and smoothly, add a loud, forceful "NO!" as you thrust forward. Yell the word, using all your lung power. Repeat this final part of the exercise three times.

Stand still, with your arms at your side, and notice the sensations in your body. People usually speak of feeling "tingling," "full of energy," "powerful." I sometimes do this exercise before going to a meeting where I expect to deal with challenging people. I do it in order to embody a clear no—not as a way to be defiant, but to fill up with a powerful energy that allows me to take a firm stand if needed. I also do one of the following exercises to establish in my body the grounding for saying yes with that same kind of clarity and authority, when that is what's called for.

Exercise: Say Yes with Your Whole Body

You can practice saying yes with your whole body as a way to generate enthusiasm, confidence, and energy. It can help you go from a ho-hum state of *Well, OK, I suppose I can do this* to *Yes, you can count on me!* Perhaps more important, you're declaring to yourself, *Yes, I can count on me.* So many decisions tend to be halfhearted. *I'll see. If I have time. If I'm in the mood.* These half-made decisions create mind clutter, a collection of unfinished business that leaves you with fractured energy that is distracting and tiring. Women often claim that men don't want to make commitments to them. But what about making commitments to yourself? That requires making a choice, a definitive yes. Even if your decision involves saying no to something or someone, that no clears the way to say yes to what you most value.

Here's how to practice entering into a state of yes. From a standing position, bend over at the waist—with knees relaxed, arms and head hanging down. Begin saying yes while slowly raising your arms and torso to bring yourself upright. Draw out the word and increase your volume as you go, eventually throwing your arms up in the air slightly behind your head and completing the word yes with full volume, like the unrestrained singing of a cardinal. You are saying yes to your decision, yes to yourself, yes to life. Feel the energy, the vitality of *living* yes with your whole body.

Exercise: Be Still and Say Yes

Saying yes can also be a quiet act. I often become still and seek clarification from my spiritual Source when I'm wavering on a decision or when my enthusiasm for something I've chosen is at half-mast. I write a question or concern on a piece of paper. Then I listen to soothing music, focus my attention on my heart, and call up feelings of love. I fill my heart with as much love as I can manage—love for myself or for someone else. Turning my attention to love brings me "home" to my Source. If my love tank feels empty, I recall an experience when I felt very loving—or felt deeply loved. I reactivate that feeling of love as much as possible.

I quiet my mind and rest in this love, trusting I will get whatever guidance I need. I give little thought to my dilemma during this period of rest and quiet. I just bask in the love.

After about fifteen minutes (you can use more or less time if you try this), I pick up pen and paper. Keeping my attention on listening to my heart's wisdom, I jot down messages or sketch images that come to me. From the stillness, from my heart, I find a thread to follow. A knowing—a yes (or no)—settles into the center of my being. I let it expand and take over my whole body. When I act from this grounded knowing birthed in stillness, I move forward confidently and passionately.

Try this exercise yourself. It's especially powerful when done in a group so that all can share out loud the guidance received. The energy of the whole group embracing silence and generating love heightens the capacity of each person to get the most of the experience. You can also use the exercise in an abbreviated form anytime during your day that you feel sluggish or stuck in indecision. With practice, you'll learn to trust the wisdom of your heart to disperse the clouds in your brain and reveal the sunshine from your Source. You'll be able to make agreements with a permeating heart-based confidence and commitment. When your whole being carries the energy of yes, you will be unstoppable.

What Does Your Body Have to Say?

OBSERVE AND REFLECT

NOTICE DECISIONS IN YOUR BODY: In the course of a day, take note of three or four significant decisions you make and how they register in your body. What body posture do you assume as you consider or carry out these decisions? Do you feel fully energized and committed to them? Does any part of your body ache or hurt when you find yourself wavering between yes and no?

GROUP "YES" AND "NO" PRACTICE: If you are part of a group, ask the group to practice the yes and no exercises in this chapter together. Then have each person practice a specific "no" they wish to say to someone. Be friendly coaches for each other by giving each woman feedback about her posture, movements, vocal quality, eye contact, and other observable activity as she speaks. If she is saying no, but her eyes are looking at the floor and you can barely hear her, invite her to take a deep breath and reconnect with the full power of the thrusting NO! and try again with eyes looking ahead and using a bigger voice. Don't criticize or push her, but lovingly encourage greater embodiment of the no she wants to say.

"No" PRACTICE: Practice saying no in front of a mirror. Say it in various ways—fearfully, brazenly, comically, in a teasing way, respectfully. Vary the volume. As you say each no, be aware of your posture, movements, facial expression, and feeling of energy. Have fun with this exercise. Use it as a warm-up for saying a no you need to say.

WRITE

REFLECTIVE JOURNALING: Journal about your observations in the above exercises.

GIVE YOUR BODY A VOICE IN DECISIONS: Give some part of your body a "voice" concerning a decision you want to make. To do this, notice some area that feels discomfort. For example, if your neck is tense, your writing might begin with: "Saying yes would be a pain in the neck because . . ." Then ask other parts of your body that are not in pain to respond, offering support—offering their yes to you. For example, your spinal cord's written comments might begin, "You can count on me to stand up straight for you, to help you hold your neck high . . ." Let the reassuring and integrating forces expressed in your various body areas serve your decision process.

LIVE

ANCHOR DECISIONS PHYSICALLY: Establish a physically anchoring activity for yourself that will help you make and follow through wholeheartedly with decisions. Then use it in your day-to-day decision-making moments. Examples include stirring up feelings of love in your heart, straightening your spine, feeling the energy in your feet, and taking a conscious breath as you move from one activity to another.

Learning from the Body of Grief

When piano movers came to take away my upright grand Chickering a few years ago, it was so heavy that three men were needed to hoist it onto the truck. They did the job quickly though, just another stop on their day's checklist. But a surprising, massive grief settled over me as I watched them drape my beloved piano with a covering and lift it like a casket. It was as if the weight of the piano settled into my torso. Even my breathing felt labored, as if each inhalation required me to lift a great many pounds.

This piano was more to me than strings, keys, and pedals in a wooden box. It held stories of my childhood—memories of my progress from "Three Blind Mice" to simplified versions of Bach and Beethoven to imagined sounds of wild applause for my "someday" performance on *The Ed Sullivan Show*. It held stories of my former husband pounding out the "Moonlight Sonata" to sweeten his sour moods and memories of my son hyperactively racing through piano practice. This piano represented a lifetime of tender moments and a collection of lost dreams. Gone now were the possibilities for my once-imagined performance career. Gone was the dream of my husband's music serenading me into old age. Gone was the promise of my son's musical future. The departure of the piano reminded me that the two people who had held my heart and shared my daily life for more than two decades were gone from my home forever.

It was the grief for all these losses that settled into my body that day. Now that the piano carrying all these unfinished stories and lost dreams had gone out the door, I was left to carry them myself. Their weight, feeling the size of the piano itself, stayed with me for days. It was only through tending to this grief, using some of the methods described in this book, that I could shed that weight and find the missing "music" inside myself.

How does grief register in your body?

Grief is a physical feeling. When we lose what we cherish, feelings of heaviness and lethargy are common. We can't think straight. Our usual aches and pains seem to get worse. Tears spring up. Or we experience more subtle signs. Things just don't feel right. We're irritated. All these feelings of grief arise to pull our attention inward so we can tend to the wounds of separation. Our body invites us to mourn. The experience can seem frightening as it takes over and wrests away our normal sense of control. Besides, it's painful.

How do you experience grief? Are you aware of it as a common emotion, happening to you many times a day? You might experience grief not just when a loved one dies or during a sad movie, but also when a friend doesn't return a phone call, a family outing is canceled, or an anticipated sale falls through. You may feel sad when a treasured item gets broken, a favorite co-worker resigns, or a visitor you enjoy leaves. To some degree, whenever something you enjoy comes to an end or whenever a dream is dashed, that's an occasion for grief. Change of any kind brings in the new and leaves behind the old. In all these situations, it's normal to experience feelings of loss.

Grief can show up even when a change is for the good. Many people who have gone through great difficulty as family caregivers grieve after the people they care for die, not only over the loss of this cherished person but also over their own status as caregiver. The days of hard work and the agony of watching someone they love suffer miserably are behind them. That's a source of relief, but then they miss being the "helper." They are no longer needed in the same way. Their role has changed. Loss of identity is a great source of grief. With aging comes a whole array of such losses—some small, some enormous.

Count the casualties—yikes!

What significant changes or losses have you experienced in the past decade?

- Hair turning gray?
- Menopause?
- Loss of physical strength, endurance, or flexibility?
- Decrease in ability to see or hear?
- Loss of mental abilities?
- Loss of skin tautness?
- Decrease in sexual desire?
- Loss of youthful appearance?
- Decrease in body moisture?
- Loss of height?
- Loss of bone density?
- Loss of "perkiness" in your breasts?
- Loss of a slim waistline?
- Loss of body parts?
- Loss of ability to sleep through the night?
- Other health losses?
- Change in work or family roles?
- Death of a dear one?
- Loss of hope?
- Loss of feelings of invulnerability?

Not all of these losses and changes relate directly to aging. Some result from genetic, environmental, or lifestyle influences. Yet the longer we live, the more susceptible we are to health decline, loss of loved ones, and other irreversible changes. Loss is so much a part of getting older that we might as well make ourselves at home in the land of grief.

Does all of this seem too depressing to think about? That makes sense. It's natural to want to feel happy and to hold on to what we value, especially our life and health. Yet loss is part of our everyday experience, and grief has a way of insisting on getting our attention. The body literally cries out for help. Sometimes, though, thinking about our losses seems overwhelming and we run away. Many addictive behaviors are an escape from grief. Alcohol or busyness or eating act as temporary salves, but the pain keeps showing up. Sometime we sink into grief and stay stuck there. One woman I met had gained forty pounds since her husband's death a year earlier. She was unable to work and was still crying several times a day. "I can't stop thinking about him," she told me. Unhealed or ignored grief can become a cancer, feeding depression, anger, and fear. Because grief is so common and so persistent, it merits a closer look if we are to age consciously.

Meet grief at the door and let it in

Oddly, the more intimate we become with grief, the less power it has over us. In this case, familiarity breeds contentment. Not that the pain of loss necessarily becomes lighter, but it enters our home as less of a stranger.

Grief usually hits closest to home when a family member becomes seriously ill. When Pam—a woman with bright eyes, a radiant smile, and long blonde hair—learned of her mother's Alzheimer's diagnosis, the news hit her especially hard. Already challenged by serious health problems of her own, including fibromyalgia and hepatitis, Pam wondered where she'd get the strength to deal with her mother's inevitable decline. Over time, as her mother's condition worsened, Pam became reluctant to visit her. "I would notice this physical stiffening in my body and this feeling of not wanting to see the pain," Pam said, demonstrating by contracting her shoulders and tucking in her chin. "I wanted to be able to communicate with her verbally."

When minds cannot connect, bodies still have a language, and Pam began to seek communion with her mother in ways that went beyond words. "One holiday, I was feeling particularly crummy with my fibromyalgia. Mother would take my hand and touch me. I laid my head down in her lap and she put her hand on my shoulder. I could feel my body relax and her body relax, and I fell asleep in her lap. I found a way to connect with her essence without the words. I let her be my mother and also let her know I was there. This was a big turning point for me."

Pam was beginning to go beyond noticing what was *gone* to treasure what was left. "On Thanksgiving, I was with her alone, and I played CDs of her favorite songs. She lit up. She sat back and closed her eyes and sang along to all the words. I could watch in her body—and in my body—this wonderful soothing. My mother said, 'It was a wonderful afternoon,' and for her to listen to this CD with Harry Belafonte on it and to watch how she rolled her eyes with sensual pleasure at thinking of him . . ." Pam stopped speaking for a while, smiling and looking far away—back to that fondly remembered moment with her mother.

"Finally, I realized that her spirit was still there. Her true nature was still there. I decided to go there and be with her true essence. All the things I loved were still there. I could feel the comfort by being around her."

As I listened to Pam's story, I found another kind of comfort in the reminder that, if I ever experience Alzheimer's, I may still retain some of my body's pleasures. In fact, old pleasures often resurface for people with dementia, their bodies still retaining memories lost to their minds.

Treasure what is left

While Pam felt comfort in retaining a connection with her mother's essence and memories, she also found another treasure: she was given a fresh eye to recognize the legacies that both her parents had passed on to her. "As my mother was dying, she started not to look like herself, and I was aware that my dad was aging too. I'd find myself looking in the mirror, trying to figure out which parts of myself looked like him and which parts looked like my mom. My forehead looks like my father, and my nose looks like my mother. Then I would think about each of their gifts. I have my father's ambition, his intellectual curiosity. My attitude of appreciation is more from my mother. I carry all that in my body too. I'm not just carrying their DNA, but the environment they gave me. The lessons I learned from my mother, I carry in my cells' memory. She'll never be gone from me."

Pam realized that the same had been true of her grandmother's legacy. "My grandmother was a gardener. Every time I plant or go to garden stores, and when I water my plants, I feel the part of her that's in me. When I plant, I feel my grandmother with me."

Think of someone precious to you who has died or left your life in some other way. Imagine yourself living inside this person's skin when she was in your life. Imagine seeing through her eyes, walking in her shoes. Try to make this experience as physically vivid as possible. How did this person laugh? How did she carry herself as she walked? What did she love to touch? How is your body like hers? How have you taken on her ways? How does this person live on in you? How could you adopt more of what you loved about her into your way of living? If you did so, imagine how you would physically feel, respond, or create your experience differently.

In the face of her mother's losses, Pam found a fresh appreciation for her ancestors' abilities and vitality and for her own—a perspective that emerged slowly, with attention to her own body, mind, and spirit. She had listened to the call of grief to slow down, to *re-view*, and she found a valuable legacy.

Accept your body as it is today

Pam's conscious attentiveness to her experiences of grief also brought to her awareness one more set of distressing losses to face. "My mother's body was changing. It was horrifying. She had always been an extremely elegant woman, dressed beautifully in jeweled tones. I was feeling dread every time I'd go to see her." Pam not only mourned her mother's decline, but she also got a glimpse of what might lie ahead for herself. "It caused me to look at the way I dress, the way *my* body was aging." Pam felt shock and grief for not only what was gone but what *will* be gone. As a woman, she knew that society is generally unforgiving and dismissive of women whose appearance falls outside of certain "beauty" norms.

As I reflect on Pam's story, I can't help but think of my own mother in her older years—with her gray hair, her wrinkled and dry skin. When I look in the mirror now, gray hairs peek through, no matter how much henna I apply. My skin is drying and wrinkling, and it is no longer clear. Assorted spots, nodules, and pockmarks *mark* me as old. These changes have been gradual, but they are becoming more pronounced. I can't deny it: I don't have the body I had ten years ago. I can't help wondering how

I will look ten or twenty years from now. Besides my mother, I have seen enough aged women to imagine what is coming. No doubt you have, too. As in Pam's case, certain moments of recognizing what's lost and what *will* be lost jar us. Grief knocks on the door again. No amount of wrinkle cream or hair color covers up what our body knows. Time is passing.

The losses are real. Yet we do not have to run and hide from them. Curiosity and courage can override any fears that arise, if you stay conscious and connected to your body, mind, and spirit through the process.

Pam stayed consciously present to her many losses. As she became aware of changes in her looks, she felt grief not only over these losses but also over her decreasing ability to move around, to work, and to think clearly because of her health problems. So many of us, in midlife, have *something* that slows us down or limits what we can do. For Pam, watching her mother deteriorate and die made her own decline more obvious to her. Yet she also viewed this circumstance with her mother as a door through the grief she felt over her own losses. "It was an opportunity to remember I was alive and that I didn't want to waste one speck of my body's vitality," she said, adding, "Whatever infirmities my body has, I'm not dying today. I can choose to embrace every moment I have." As result, said Pam, "I've been more accepting. Instead of wanting my body to be what it was, I'm accepting what it is. As I accept me now, I don't have to define myself as not what I used to be."

Accepting ourselves as we are now, as Pam describes, is not the same as defining ourselves by our diseases. Yet we tend to do that. We speak of "my arthritis" or "my heart problem," and before long our condition merges with our self-definition. When asked, "How are you?" we respond with, "Well, my arthritis is . . . ," followed by an update on whether the condition has gotten better or worse.

Do you have chronic health problems that tend to define you? How else could you define yourself? What are your body's strengths? What have you *found* even in the midst of your losses?

Sometimes, salient metaphors can be our guides into the land of loss. While dryness, graying hair, sagging skin, and other signs of aging are generally considered undesirable, dried plants (some quite wrinkled) are considered beautiful, and a silver color is considered attractive in jewelry.

James Hillman, in *The Force of Character and the Lasting Life*, reminds us of our role as the light bearers and wise ones in our community, requiring sufficient dryness to kindle a flame and to crystallize into the salt of the earth. His book offers a rich array of archetypal images and a good deal of wit in suggesting such refreshing takes on the many bodily changes that come with aging. What other comparisons can you come up with that can help you find a wider range of appreciation for the changing aspects of your body?

Heal the old grief and the new

Grief is often as much about past losses as it is about current ones. Haven't you gone to a memorial service and found yourself feeling sadness about a loved one who died long ago even as you listened to the eulogy and words of comfort concerning the person who has just died? Often we move through periods of loss in our life without adequate opportunities to grieve, and the grief stays lodged in our heart or throat or elsewhere in our body. It can show up unprovoked years later. The longer we live, the more of this unexpressed grief we accumulate. I've had times when I've welcomed a chance to go to a funeral because I'd been feeling a lot of sadness over a series of losses or disappointments in my life and wanted an outlet for it, a chance to cry openly.

Some grief may be very old, still simmering from losses as far back as our childhood. My father's suicide when I was eight left me with a legacy of grief, not so much from the death itself but from the gap it created in growing up without the strength of my dad to back me up when I needed to be strong. It was only in my late fifties, with the help of a bodyworker, that I tapped into that sadness, which I carried in my lower back. As I did, I felt as if I were eight years old again, longing for my dad's presence. At the prompting of the bodyworker, I spoke to the spirit of my dad and told him how hard it was to miss out on the kind of security and backup I needed. Then I felt a very strong sense of the presence of my father immediately standing behind me, and what happened then I can only describe as a merging of his presence, his strength, into my backbone. I finally felt that at last I had "backup."

What old sadness do you carry inside you? Where does it reside in your body? Try asking your body to show you any unhealed grief.

Whether you're dealing with current or old grief, you can take steps to move through the grief by honoring what your body requires.

Exercises: Feeling Your Grief

1. Acknowledge the loss. You don't have to tough it out, pretend it isn't happening, or try to cover it up. In Pam's case, she admitted the loss of her mother's abilities and her changes in appearance, and she reflected on her own body's losses as well.

2. Let the grief surface. Cultural taboos against expressing grief beyond a few tears are so strong that most of us have learned to keep our sorrow under wraps or think we should get over it quickly. In addition, mixed in with grief can be anger, relief, tenderness, and other feelings. It may not be so important to sort out all the feelings as to let them arise. Notice where in your body you're feeling something different from your everyday feelings—a tiredness, a heavy heart, difficulty with swallowing. It may be only a subtle sign of grief—less interest in your favorite foods, a curling of your hands into fists, or some way of pursing your lips or holding your jaw. Each of us has a unique way to inhabit our grief. Pam noticed herself stiffening up when she went to visit her mother, a sign of her resistance to the losses. This was the beginning of the grieving process for her.

3. Give yourself some prompts. If you can't readily identify or feel the grief, start writing with "What I miss most about _____ is _____" or "If I were sad, it would be about _____." Rituals such as prayers or candle lighting can also help prompt your grief to open up. Put yourself physically near a person or situation that will activate the grief. Another option is to put on some mournful or tender music to arouse emotion, or you can curl up in a rocking chair and rock yourself as a mother might rock her child. When

using these prompts, pay close attention to how your body is reacting.

4. Let your body lead you. If you feel like singing a sad song, sing
   it. If you feel like curling up, do so—and stay curled up until you
   feel an urge to do something else. Rhythmic moving can be very
   comforting, so notice if any part of you wants to sway or roll. Pam
   relaxed in her mother's lap as a way to settle into her grief and find
   its tender side. Pay special attention to any sounds that emerge.
   If you sigh, sigh again and sigh bigger. Let moaning sounds come
   out. Grieving does not have to be contained. Wail loud and long.
   Let it all out. Take your time.

5. Create a closing ritual. It could be as simple as saying or writing
   a prayer, dedicating yourself to something meaningful related to
   your loss, or discarding something as a sign of change or completion. Pam said she "had to clear out anything that looked like
   Alzheimer's out of the house, so just the reminders of my mother's
   spirit could be present." At a wake I attended, a green ribbon
   (green for hope) was unfurled and passed among us. Each person
   taking hold of the ribbon spoke of personal memories of the de-
   ceased, and having the ribbon in our hands united all of us present in our love for her and in our grief. Then, a scissors was passed
   around, so we could each cut a piece of the ribbon to take home
   as a remembrance of her. Such a ritual helps to bring closure to
   this period of grief and signals a readiness to move on. It's also a
   celebration of grief as a healing emotion.

Swirl into a dance of grief

During a recent summer, tornado winds swept through the neighborhood
where I live, taking out power and leaving more than ten thousand trees
in the area bent, split, or prone. On a walk through a nearby park preserve
the next morning, I had to climb under or over fallen trees about every fifty
yards. In my own yard, two tall pines lay stretched out. And around a large
pond behind my home, two willows gave in to the wind and their branches lay strewn helplessly across the water. The trunk of one willow, so big

around that three sets of extended arms might be needed to reach around its girth, was bent and torn open like a large piece of cracked celery.

Something in my chest felt split and broken open as I drifted among this wasteland of devastated trees. I love trees, especially tall ones. When I stand or walk among them, I feel tall, able to reach up and out. In their presence, I trust in beauty and longevity. My spirit feels full. I know that all is right with the world and with me.

Losing so many of these sure and beautiful green monuments to life left me feeling sluggish, dazed, less sure. A big piece of the life I love had been whooshed away, out of my control. For the next few days, I often sat on a fallen branch in my back yard, stunned into unrushed silence amidst the emptied space around me and in the empty space in my heart. I craved stillness. I sat, barely breathing, in silent homage, keeping watch until the fallen trees could be taken away. After a time, I noticed that the falling of the trees had opened up the view around me. I was less closed off from my neighbors. More light was coming in, giving pleasure to my eyes. Meantime, the electrical power in the area was being restored.

After this extended time of quietly sitting with the devastation, at last I felt like dancing the story of this loss and restoration, and later that week in my Free Motion group, I did. I twirled and swirled with the memory of the winds propelling me. I swung back and forth with the resilience of those trees that had enough give in their branches to withstand the force of the tornado winds. I danced cracking and splitting motions and falling to the ground. I celebrated with open arms and scanning gaze the expanded view to the horizon and a rebirth of power.

What Does Your Body Have to Say?

OBSERVE AND REFLECT

SPEND TIME WITH LOSS: Spend time with someone who is older and has lost some abilities. Notice your own physical reactions around this person. Where do you feel tense or ill at ease? What do you notice your hands doing? What's happening in your belly? In your chest?

NOTICE WHAT'S LEFT: Spend time with another such person. This time give your attention to what's "left." Take note of the person's capabilities. Observe compensating activities, such as a blind person's acute hearing.

WRITE

THANKS FOR THE LOSS: Make a list of your losses in recent years. Make a check mark by each one that feels unfinished. For each checked loss, write a thank-you letter for the gifts you carry within you from that person, object, or situation. Even if all you can think of are treasured memories, express thanks for those. You can address the letter to the person, object, or situation; address it to your Source; or write it to yourself in acknowledgement of attracting and enjoying this particular treasure in your life.

LIVE

GROUP HONORING OF GRIEF: Gather with a group of women friends for a time of grief honoring. Invite each woman to bring a symbol of what she has lost. Create a ritual setting with candles, soft cloths, ribbons, or other items that support a nurturing and sacred environment. Open the circle of grief with music, singing a welcoming song or chanting together. Then let each woman tell her story of loss verbally or nonverbally. Offer your open arms and heart to each other. Be a hearth of love and compassion for one another. But let each woman have her own grief and feel it fully. Your job is not to take it away but to be a circle of compassionate witnesses. Have faith in each woman's capacity to grieve and to heal. When all have finished, use a song, chant, or dance to complete the circle of grief and bring the ritual to a close.

DAILY RHYTHMS OF GRIEF: In your daily life, pay attention to losses as they arise. Feel your grief, welcome it. Notice where it resides in your body. Let it arise, have its say, and move through you. Remember that loss and grief are part of the natural rhythm of your days.

COMMUNITY GRIEF SUPPORT: Consider attending grief groups, workshops, or retreats that many hospices, hospitals, and faith communities offer to support people through times of loss. The compassion and guidance you find there may allow you to safely cry, create rituals, or use other means to express and process your grief.

CHAPTER 12

Writing from Your Body

When I tell women in their fifties or older that I write books, their first response is often an enthusiastic "Really? That's something *I* want to do." Women who have lived awhile have stories to tell. They want to let other people know what it felt like to be called ugly in tenth grade, get promoted when no one thought they could, bury their children or lovers, rise up in the face of addiction or cancer, or run for office. By making a written record of their lives, women fulfill a creative urge.

But there's more at stake. They want to leave a legacy in order to confirm that their lives have had meaning and to pass along the wisdom they've acquired. Some of them hope to find added meaning and wisdom as they write.

Have you written your story? Or, I should say, "stories." Chances are you've lived a lifetime filled with experiences worth writing about. Getting them on paper instills new life into them. Sharing them with others gives them wings.

But where to start? How can you put on paper the significant experiences of your life in a way that conveys more than facts? How can you capture your stories' grit and grace?

Use details to tell your story

"Tell the truth," an early writing teacher of mine taught me. The way to do that, I learned, was by using vivid details. Rather than writing "I walked to school after missing the bus," include sounds, colors, tempo, or other particulars: "The heels of my shiny white shoes clicked on the sidewalk like a metronome's rapid tick-tock, matching my heart rate, as I raced to arrive at school before the last bell rang." As a reader of such writing, my senses are tickled. The scene comes to life. I am *there* with the writer. By the same token, the writing comes alive for the writer. The more details I call to mind and use when writing my stories, the more alive I feel. More of me is *there* as I reactivate my physical sensations from the experience. In this kind of vivid writing, the exchange between reader and writer becomes an intimate exchange, because both people are fully present.

Use sensory memory to recall the details

As you recollect your experiences in preparation for writing about them, let your senses serve as tour guides through your memories. What did you see, hear, touch, smell, or taste? Did you hear the snap of the light switch, the pop and hiss of the champagne bottle being opened, the key turning in the lock? Was it the aroma of burnt beans, pumpkin pie, or fried fish that greeted you when you came on the scene?

Exercise: Active Reminiscing

To help you remember, try Active Reminiscing. Close your eyes and imagine re-entering the setting where your story takes place. Bring yourself back into the experience as fully as you can by reactivating the physical sensations you had at the time. (Before recalling a highly traumatic situation, you may wish to seek the assistance of a professional or find other support.) What are you touching? Of all the things within your view, where are your eyes focused? What or who is making noise?

Go beyond the usual five senses, and settle into your visceral feelings. Is your gut churning, or has anger given you an adrenaline rush? Are you filled with energy or feeling sluggish? Notice how warm or cold your body is. Do you feel any discomfort? What about your physical position and posture? Are you standing or sitting upright? Is there any weight or pressure on your body? What parts of you, if any, are moving?

As you revisit your experiences in memory, open your eyes from time to time and jot down as many details as you can. *Grape jelly on his face. Her humped shoulders and sunken chest. My bunions throbbing. Cinnamon candle scent. My parents whispering their argument in the hallway. Sneezing from the wheat chaff up my nose. Curled lips and tight larynx, holding back a scream.* Put on paper anything that comes to your mind—or maybe I should say, anything that comes to your body. To further prompt your writing, ask your various body parts for help: Belly, what was going on inside of you at the time? Legs, how fast did you want to move? Jaw, what did you think of the situation? The more you can recall and jot down your physical sensations and reactions, the more specific language you'll have to invite your readers inside the situation alongside you. Then you'll be able to help them understand what you understood, feel what you felt.

Use analogies and sensory prompts

Another way to add vivid sensory detail to your writing is through analogies. *He stood stiff and still as a fence post. I picked up the knitting needles as if they were made of lead. Her face softened like butter.* Comparisons help readers understand your experience by relating it to something they're familiar with. To make analogies, tap into your body memories. Let's say you want to describe the quality of the sound of someone's voice; your ears have a huge library of sound recordings you can use for comparison. What *else* have you heard that sounds like this voice? A scraper removing winter ice from a windshield? A child's whining? The pitch of a teapot whistle?

If you need further help recalling the kind of details that will make your writing vibrant, use sensory prompts. Pull out old photos or objects related to the topic you want to write about. Burn a candle with a scent reminiscent of the experience. Return to the sights and sounds of the experience if possible. Go back to the health club where you met your one great love and let the sauna there heat up your memories. Revisit the mountain trail where you had to be carried down by rescuers so you can describe well the sweetness of the huckleberries that one of them picked for you along the way. If you can't physically return to the nursing home where you held your mother's hand as she died, walk the halls of a similar nursing home to refamiliarize you with the wide aisles, the crooked-tooth smiles, and the walkers with tennis balls on the legs.

As you go on these sensory adventures, record the details in a notebook, on your laptop, or on an audio recorder. With this record at hand as you write your story, you'll have images and language that invite the reader to accompany you on your memory trail. You may make some new discoveries as well.

When I was getting ready to write the final chapter of *Body Odyssey*, on illness and death, I felt at a loss for how to talk about death. Although I'd had plenty of experience with illness, I hadn't had to confront death closely myself nor had I spent much time with people dying. The topic felt so remote to me at that time that I wasn't sure I could write about it with much sensitivity.

One day, looking through a closet, I happened upon a box of memorabilia from Sister Pat, my sister who was a Catholic nun and who had died twenty years earlier, in her fifties. The box held writings and photos of her, as well a few plastic statues and holy cards she had given me. Touching and looking at these items washed up a river of grief and a flood of memories associated with her life and death. I got just what I needed to write the chapter.

Once I'd found the box in the closet, I entered into Active Reminiscing, stepping back in time to when I sat beside Sister Pat near the time of her death, recalling the sights, sounds, and feelings there as fully as I could. I reexperienced the melting warmth my heart felt as I looked at the softened quality of her body lying in front of me. When Sister Pat had helped to raise me in my preschool years (her name was Lucille then), she had always seemed so rigid. With her stiff jaw and scolding brow, she had corralled me into rigid obedience. My child body and demeanor had stiffened to match hers in order to win her authoritative, approving smile. But now, cancer's ravages and her deep surrender to love and to God had altered the quality of her body. It bore no signs of tightness in her jaw or elsewhere. She had told me a few weeks earlier that her biggest regret was that she had not learned to love earlier. Now, her kind eyes, reassuring voice, and soft jaw spoke of nothing but love.

I made many notes as I returned in memory to these experiences. By relying on these notes *and by returning to the state of Active Reminiscence* when it came time to write my chapter on death, I was easily able to invite readers into what I was witnessing and discovering at my sister's deathbed. Here's what I wrote about the influence of Sister Pat's early "mothering" on me: "I became a good girl, too, obeying the rules and faithfully tucking my true feelings and desires into my tense jaw, shoulders, hips, and other pseudo-safe places. As with her, my ingratiating smile over a stern demeanor and my hard-work ethic were, for so many years, what I thought I needed in order to be pleasing, to be loved, to get it 'right.'" As I shared this moment of personal insight and vulnerability, I gave readers a close-up tour of my thoughts and physical sensations, helping them feel at home with me.

I also described what I saw as I looked at my sister lying there in front of me: "Her furrow-browed scold was gone. Her jaw seemed at ease." As I recalled seeing this changed face, I reflected on what might be my own physical and spiritual state when it's my time to die: "As I sat watching her breathe during my final visit, I wondered, is this how it will be in the end for me—tensions worn down, shapes softened, ragged as the Velveteen Rabbit?"

All this remembering, reflecting, and writing came from touching the objects she gave me, from reading her writings, and from allowing myself to return to the somatic experiences of that final time with her. My body opened the gate to a private estate of memories, resulting in writing that conveyed vibrancy and meaning.

While the topic of my stories was the body itself, the practices of Active Reminiscing and heightened somatic awareness can bring a visceral realness to stories on any topic. What experiences do you want to write about? Put pen in hand, settle back in your chair, and let your body memories take you to a starting place.

Let your body tell the story

If your ears could describe what they've heard and how it affected them, what would they say? Try asking them. Writing the history of a *particular area of your body* can be another way to explore your body wisdom and share your learning with others. Let that body area become the storyteller.

Let's say you have a scar on your body and you want to tell the story of how you got it and the lessons you learned. Trust your scar to do the talking.

In my journal, around the time my (unplanned) son left home to go to college, I let the stretch marks on my belly write to me of their wisdom—wisdom I particularly needed to be reminded of at that time:

I am the mother scar, the marks that let your womb make room for a son to rise within you. I came to teach you about loving what you could not control and the lesson is not over yet. You had to give yourself over to me once and let me have my way. I stretched you beyond where you wanted to go, beyond where you thought you could go. You had no mothering in you, so you had to make it up, create an opening for it, find the maternal mystery. You are still being stretched, as your body and your whole life change with age, and as your son now leaves home. You can go into it, let it take you. It does not matter if your belly changes shape or you have more scars to wear. Imagine what new son may be rising within you that you cannot control. Imagine how it may bless you.

What areas of your body have interesting histories? What might they tell you if you put a pen in their "hand"?

Write your sexual history

Our sexual organs are a rich but often overlooked source of stories about our experiences as women. Consider writing your sexual history.

Not long ago, a friend in her fifties told me the history of her most significant sexual experiences. She had put in it writing, and now she wanted someone who cared about her to hear and understand what she'd endured, lost, and discovered through several sexual incidents that left long-standing wounds. I'm not going to discuss the details of her revealing and painful story, but I will tell you it touched me deeply. I felt honored to be trusted with this intimate act of friendship, which brought us closer than ever.

As I looked back on that conversation, I was also surprised to realize how rarely I have had such a get-real conversation with a friend about personal sexual experiences. In talking with other women, I learned that such conversations are indeed rare. Isn't it odd that we keep so much of our sexual life a secret? The social taboos against talking about sex in more than a flippant way are huge.

In correspondence I received from Evelyn Beck, PhD, a retired professor of women's studies at the University of Maryland, she reminded me that "historically, a 'good' woman was taught to be a prude" and that "women have been taught NOT to have desire or sexual pleasure." She continued, "Even now, after the 'sexual revolution,' many men still prefer women to be responsive [and not] the initiators. Women who really want their own pleasure are often seen as not a 'good' woman. In Victorian times, women were called 'the sex,' as if only women carried the mark of gender, but they were NOT to be sexual. I think even today, many women are afraid to own their own desire and are afraid to admit to wanting pleasure, perhaps even to themselves." Beck added that "lesbians or bisexual women may be particularly terrified of their own sexuality, since it is likely that they were brought up to believe that same sex desire or love is wrong. This would be especially true for older women who came out at a time when same-sex relationships had to be hidden. Historically, same-sex love was seen as sin, sickness, or a crime, and in spite of recent changes in public attitudes, many women, old and young, still suffer from these fears of stigma."

No wonder, then, that our sexual stories remain so secretive. Many women never reveal their history of sexual abuse that left them feeling ashamed, angry, and confused. Others do their best to ignore the residue of miscarriages, stillbirths, and abortions. Many older women long to be held and caressed but have no one available, and they're afraid to let anyone know about their desires. Still others have a great sex life that stays a secret outside their intimate relationship. Some women worry that they're not doing sex the "right" way or often enough. They rely on Oprah's advice (a wise woman, to be sure) and movie images as their guides, but they miss out on the self-discovered wisdom that emerges in honest personal conversations with trusted friends. I think it's safe to say that a great many women seldom talk directly about the subject of sex except in a humorous or clinical way.

How much of your sexual story have you explored in any depth? How much have you kept secret out of shame or fear?

The menopausal years are an ideal time to do a comprehensive personal sexual review—and possibly share it with women friends, your partner, or someone else you trust. These years are a time when your sexual interests may be changing, and you're confronted with some very real losses: your breasts may sag, your vaginal juices diminish, and your response to stimulation slows down. Still, you can continue to be a passionate woman with a lust for pleasure. Masturbation and sexual toys made for women can generate your enjoyment alone and may even help you discover more about what you find pleasurable—once-forbidden territory for women. Also, as Connie Goldman so wonderfully illustrates through interviews with older couples in *Late-Life Love: Romance and New Relationships in Later Years,* the pleasures of sex with a partner can continue into the eighties and beyond.

After I divorced in my late forties, I was very surprised by a new relationship that sparked intense sexual feelings. My new partner and I spent every spare minute making love. My fire was definitely not out. It was invigorating to feel the romantic high, and I found myself walking and talking in a more sensual manner overall. I suspect this kind of refiring is fairly common in a midlife romance after the painful years of a failing marriage. But I was particularly intrigued by the physical differences that were evident in my day-to-day life. I literally looked, moved, and sounded different. My movements were more fluid, I had a softer smile, and my voice had a lilting, alluring tone to it. Sex had a softening, enlivening effect on me.

Even if sexual interest goes on simmer or shuts off, that's not the end of a woman's femininity. And whether we have a partner in later years or not, we are still sensual beings capable of maintaining fluid softness and sensuous voices. But our anatomy is changing and we do feel and think differently. Women I've talked to speak of feeling relief that their hormones are not running their lives the way they used to, allowing them to relate to other people with more clarity and fewer sexual overtones. Many women are glad to be through with the messiness and crampiness of their periods, while others miss the monthly reminder of their fertility.

How are you responding to these changes in your body? What might you have to learn from your past and from the present realities that face you?

EXERCISE: WRITE YOUR SEXUAL HISTORY

Consider writing your sexual history as a way to celebrate what you've enjoyed, mourn what you've lost, and make peace with your past. Taking an inventory of your past and present sexual attitudes and experiences will help you clarify how and why you have developed the sexual patterns and attitudes you have. It can lead to compassion for what you've been through, appreciation for your courage along the way, and a readiness for what lies ahead. You may find a way to give yourself permission to release sexual behaviors and lingering shame that no longer serve you. You may also call up a lot of pleasant memories. Writing your sexual memoir can also prepare you to initiate conversations with your partner or with trusted friends in order to seek their understanding and insights—or their help if there is a need to forgive yourself. Depending on your experiences and how you feel about them, it could also lead to a lot of laughs.

For some women, exploring this history might seem difficult. So much shame and secrecy is associated with sexuality that it may not be an easy subject to probe. Before you begin, create a safe and nurturing environment for yourself. Treat yourself the same way you would treat a good friend who wants to tell you something very personal and important. Give yourself plenty of time to do this writing without interruption. You may even do it over several days or weeks, a half hour or more per time. Each time you work on it, put on comforting music, light a candle, wrap yourself in your comforter, or do whatever helps you feel at ease. Give special attention to the sexual areas of your body, and ask them to help you tell their story.

Here are some questions to get you started on your sexual autobiography:

1. When did you first feel sexual urges? What were the feelings that arose? Where did you feel them?

2. Who was the first person you felt an attraction to? Describe the attributes that got you excited.

3. How did you learn about sex? Recall the sensations in your body as you heard about the sex act.

4. What were some of the early messages you got about sex? From whom?

5. What effects were there from any misinformation you received?

6. What, if any, early experiences with sex were unpleasant, or even abusive? (If any feelings come up that feel too big to handle alone, be sure to get the support of caring friends or professionals.)

7. What do you remember about the first time you really knew you were a woman? Where did you feel that knowing in your body?

8. What happened when you had your first menstrual cycle? How did your body respond during your time of menses?

9. When was your sexual orientation clear to you? Did you ever have doubts about your sexual orientation? About whether you were actually female?

10. What are the values you hold about sex? How do your activities reflect, or conflict with, those values? If there are conflicts, where do those conflicts reside in your body?

11. Describe any experiences of ridicule, rejection, or betrayal you had relating to your sexuality, and how they affected you. Where did you feel those responses in your body?

12. What were some of the best sexual encounters you ever had? What made them special? Describe the feelings you had.

13. What regrets, if any, do you have about your sexual history? In what ways have you been critical of yourself for your sexual past and held on to shame about it? Where does the regret, criticism, or shame reside in your body?

14. What resentments about sexual partners are you holding onto? Where do you feel those in your body?

15. How have your sexual interests and activities changed as you've gotten older?

16. What do you miss, if anything, about what is no longer the same? Describe any sadness you feel.

17. What do you welcome about the changes you're experiencing?

18. If you don't have a partner, what does it mean to be a sexual woman at this time in your life? What does it mean if you do have a partner?

19. What do you enjoy about your sex life currently? How could you make it more satisfying?

20. What have you learned about yourself and others from your sexual experiences?

When you're through writing your history, celebrate in some way. Sketch, paint, or create a collage to give your discoveries visual expression. Do a dance that tells your story or expresses your feelings about it. Make up a song blessing yourself as a sexually vibrant woman. Then, decide if you want to share any of your history or your creations with your partner, women's group, or other trusted friends. If you do, ask them to honor what you share with respect and confidentiality.

In your inventory, you may have discovered old hurts in need of healing. Lingering shame, fear, or resentments may be camping out in your mind and body, even making you sick. Use some of the techniques you've learned in this book to help you heal. If you need further help, work with a counselor, spiritual teacher, drama or dance therapist, bodyworker, or other professional to help you heal the past and free you to enjoy your sexual nature in the years to come.

You can write a similar history about any aspect of your body's life. Perhaps you've had a long-standing health problem, and you want to tell that story. Maybe your body has an outstanding feature, such as being especially tall or beautiful or obese, that has shaped your life significantly. Putting your story on paper will help you gain clarity about its meaning. If you choose to share it with others, your story may help them gain insight into their own somatic history.

Write an opinion piece on your body

Remember when you turned forty? Was that the time you started getting the "you're so old" birthday cards? Or maybe that didn't happen until you hit forty-five or fifty. Sadly, ridicule of old age is a mainstay of the greeting card industry. But birthdays do remind us of our mortality and the passing of years. They give us milestones to reflect on our life and set ourselves on a new course. Usually, they also cause us to look in the mirror and check out the condition of our body. Here's a short essay written by a woman named Annie Kemp on one of her significant birthdays.

On Turning 45

It's almost 3 A.M. in the morning and today is my birthday. I am officially forty-five years old. Whenever I think of age, I recall Jane Fonda turning fifty and saying, "This is what fifty looks like for me and that is what fifty looks like for her and so on." It occurred to me that I have spent the majority of the first half of my life avoiding mirrors. I grew up in a time when beauty was defined in terms that I could not possibly meet, but that didn't stop me from trying. Like Whoopi Goldberg, I wrapped towels around my head to get a sense of what long hair felt like. Like my schoolmates, I tried Dippity-do in my painfully short hair with brush rollers and wound up having to cut most of my hair off to get the curlers out. I washed and scrubbed my face daily and nightly in the fervent hope I would wake up as beautiful as the women in the magazines that professed to define the terms of beauty for me.

There were only two times in my life that I was "thin" and therefore supposedly more attractive. One was when I was homeless and living on the streets. The other was during my first marriage when I became convinced that my weight was the problem and solving that problem would save my marriage. I was wrong. For forty-five years I have rejected this body I was given, although for the majority of those years it never let me down. This body carried me through four childbirths with two children who lived. It carried me through floors scrubbed on my hands and knees, working night shifts, going to college all day and living on two hours sleep. This body rocked babies to sleep against its softness, comforted a heartbroken teenage girl, and allowed a man child to break down when his daughter was moved to Florida along with her mother.

Yet for all that and more, I have hated this body endlessly. It was too fat, too short; it didn't have enough stamina, wasn't sexy, was too utilitarian. It was the kind of body that inspired men to think of me as their "buddy." I tried disguises—stretch pants and big loose shirts. It worked until I walked past a window one day and didn't recognize the woman staring back at me. Slowly and painstakingly, I began to fight against the hundreds of messages I'd been given. Baby steps, one at a time—learning to be comfortable with a hairdresser, discovering the fashion industry has finally realized large women have money too, discovering makeup and perfume at the age of forty-two. I transformed myself into the quintessential professional woman, a sophisticated external package. Yet I continued to avoid things as critical as a mammogram because it would necessitate my taking off the "costume" and being seen as I still knew I truly was—ugly.

So for my forty-fifth year on this earth, I have pledged to myself that I shall accept this body I have been given. There is not a wrinkle on my face thanks to melatonin and good genes. My teeth are as crooked now as they were when I was ten years old. I am still pear-shaped. My breasts no longer reach toward the sun, but they are still a soft place for a weary head or a broken heart to rest upon. My skin remains astonishingly soft and my touch has gentled with time and self-confidence. I can still do a perfect ballerina point with both feet as long as I'm sitting in my wheelchair. My arms are strong from pushing the chair as well as from years of use. Despite my large size, my small hands, slender wrists, and tiny feet continue to baffle me as well as make me smile.

It is the forty-fifth year of my life. I am, as they say, officially halfway there. I feel as if I spent my twenties making mistakes and my thirties making repairs. My forties seem to be about finding a level of peace within myself, first intellectually and now physically. This is who I am—soft, gentle, shy, capable of standing my ground on another's behalf. I am a passionate lover, a learning-to-be-loving mother and grandmother, and a new wife, all at the same time. I am a quilter, a writer, a research analyst.

For all this and more, this is what forty-five looks like on me, and I am pleased.

....

What does your current age look like on you? Are you pleased? Maybe it's time to write your thoughts about how your body strikes you at this time in your life. You don't have to wait for a significant birthday to pay tribute to your body, past and present.

What Does Your Body Have to Say?

OBSERVE AND REFLECT

JOURNAL REVIEW OF SEXUAL EXPERIENCES: Perhaps you have written about your sexual experiences in your journals over time. Review these journal entries. What themes emerge? What feels unfinished? Is there anyone, yourself included, whom you need to forgive or to appreciate?

WRITE

FIND A STORY IN YOUR BODY: Scan your body, looking for a good story. When you find an area of your body that has an interesting history, imagine curling up in your favorite chair and listening to it tell you a story. Write it down. What other experiences have you had that you've always wanted to write about? Start writing.

MEMOIR RESEARCH: If you want to write a complete memoir, begin keeping a story journal in which you jot down memories or ideas you want to include. Once you've jotted some things down, be alert in your day-to-day life of experiences that might serve as research opportunities for the details associated with your memories or ideas. Let's say you want to include something about a grandmother who loved to garden. When you visit a garden, nursery, or florist, take note of details about fragrances, color hues, shapes, and sizes of plants that your grandmother might have grown. Also notice if any more memories about your grandmother come up as you place yourself physically in a setting reminiscent of her environment. Jot down those details in your journal for later use when you write about her in your memoir.

LIVE

WHOLE-BODIED WRITING: Let the act of writing itself be a whole-bodied experience. As you sit down to write, relax and take a deep breath. Relax your eyes, your jaw, your shoulders, your hands. Feel yourself taking up space and being well supported in your chair. Feel how your whole body is connected to your hands as you write. Stop periodically as you write to make sure you're in your body, and that you're treating it kindly.

Your Body as a Window to the Spirit

Have you ever had a moment that felt "divine"? I'm talking about experiences of the transcendent, when you felt deeply aware of something or someone spiritual. Mystics, saints, and healers of various faith and cultural traditions see visions from other dimensions and hear directly the words of God, the Great Spirit, or other nonhuman guides. Most of us don't have such an obvious direct line to the divine. But all of us can have moments where we step outside the ordinary and become immersed in a profound experience of union with all that is.

If you're a mother, you may have had times when you were so moved by the miracle of your baby coming into being that you felt as if life and you and your child were all one continuous marvel. Wholehearted, wholebodied lovemaking, when you surrender yourself into union with another, may sweep you into an ecstasy of oneness beyond the physical. In the moments right before or after a loved one's death, you may see or feel or simply *know* the presence of beings who live on the other side. The dying themselves often speak of moving toward light and of angels or family members awaiting them.

One reason we can touch the transcendent is because the body is a window to the spirit. The more aware and present we are in our body, the wider these windows open. Many stories and exercises in both *Body Odyssey* and this book illustrate this link between flesh and spirit. You may recall, for example, Myrtle Fillmore's cure from tuberculosis after she tuned in to the God-life in her cells, described in chapter 6, and the healing pathway of stillness or silence also discussed in that chapter. This chapter will explore even more ways to deepen this body-spirit bond.

Create the intention

Our thoughts are powerful. What we think about, we create. If you start your day assuming, "This is going to be a great day," the odds are very good that some great things will happen. By contrast, if you're thinking, "I dread this day," the day is more likely to be dreadful, a reflection of your ominous thoughts.

Another way to describe the power of our thinking is to say that our thoughts are prayers. The words or images we hold in our mind reflect our beliefs. They're faith statements. What we envision, think about, feel strongly about, and declare comes into being. We create our world. This is more than a nice idea. Dr. Emoto's work with water crystals (see chapter 2) illustrates dramatically that we literally influence our environment through our thoughts and intentions. We don't know exactly how this works or why sometimes results are more quickly realized or apparent than others. But the disciplined mind has proven to be an effective creator, as demonstrated by thousands of ordinary people who have participated in firewalking—walking barefoot across fiery coals—without being burned.

So, how can you use the creative power of your mind to mingle body and spirit? Begin with intention. How would you like your body to speak to you of the spiritual realm? In truth, your body, mind, and spirit are already more closely bound than the hydrogen and oxygen that combine to form water droplets. Plunge yourself deeply into this union, declaring your readiness to learn its secrets. Open yourself to the awareness that your body is spirit in action.

Here are some affirmations you can use to declare your intention as you start your day or as you enter into a special time set aside for personal self-discovery and spiritual enrichment:

- My body is a vibrant channel for Spirit.
- I am open to touching the divine through my body.
- I am aware of Goddess energy flowing through my every cell.

Notice that these intentions are not stated as petitions or wishes. They are declarations of a fundamental belief in the presence of the divine, alive and acting through you in physical form. If thoughts (beliefs) create our reality, then setting your intentions on a foundation of affirmative thought is a good place to start. Rather than waiting to see if what you desire shows up before you believe it's there, *believe* in it in order to create it.

Stay intentional—conscious—throughout your day. Whenever your body is having a response to your circumstances, make the assumption that your spiritual nature is at work. Become curious and mindful, welcoming the chance to understand and value the spiritual forces that are dancing in your body.

A few years ago, when I had some health problems, a friend suggested I go to see Rosita, a woman who did healing work in her home. Rosita had been trained by Chunyi Lin, a Chinese qigong master, whose work I knew and who had a reputation for relieving people of serious illnesses. Qigong masters are reputed to have remarkable abilities to know and adjust what is happening in people's energy fields through highly developed sensitivity to the body's energy systems. Rosita had been healed by Master Lin of a lung condition that Mayo Clinic doctors had told her would require her to use a respiratory ventilator for the rest of her life. After Lin worked on her, she no longer needed this machine and its tubes, which she had dragged around with her for years. In gratitude for her healing, Rosita invited people with health problems into her tiny kitchen, and there she used the healing skills she had learned from Master Lin.

When I visited her home, the black-haired woman greeted me with laughter and a thick Mexican accent. I made my way to her kitchen by way of her small living room, which was crowded with images of the Guadalupe Virgin Mary and Jesus, rosaries, and Day of the Dead shrines. As I sat at her kitchen table drinking tea, Rosita stood behind me with her hands placed near my shoulders, applying her skills. I asked her to tell me how she knew what to do to help someone. "I do what Master Lin showed me," was her matter-of-fact reply. "When I'm not sure what to do, I ask Master Lin." Knowing that Master Lin was currently in China, I responded, "You call him in China and ask him?" "I don't need to call him," she said. "I just ask him." She went on to explain that she had recently been trying to help a woman with cancer but wasn't clear what to do. She was confident Master Lin would let her know. "On Sunday I went to Mass," she explained. "I was walking down the aisle to my pew, and I saw Master Lin coming toward me. Then I knew what to do for this woman with her cancer."

Rosita's clear confidence in her teacher's guidance is an inspiring example of living with declared intention. Not concerned with supposed limits of time and space, she created what was needed by expecting to receive it. Clearly, both Rosita and Master Lin had refined their ability to live in mind-body-spirit harmony. You have that ability, too. Develop it further by declaring and wholeheartedly expecting to receive what you want.

You can do this in small, everyday matters and in big affairs. Try it. Some morning, align yourself with your divine Source or guidance through prayer, meditation, or whatever form you find works well for you. Declare with conviction and enthusiasm that the perfect ideas, people, and resources will show up to help you get a specific personal or work project completed with ease. Envision the project finished in its best possible form, and start feeling the good feelings you expect to have when it's done. Look for what's going "right" throughout the day and maintain confidence that the project is moving along successfully. Be on the lookout for all the ways the universe (or God, Goddess, Allah, Source) delivers help to get the job done. No matter what may go "wrong," stay committed wholeheartedly to your vision. Remember: your thoughts are prayers with creative powers. Watch for miraculous results!

Make use of rituals

For thousands of years, people of faith have relied on rituals to activate and express their beliefs. Praying with beads, lighting candles, kneeling and prostrating, fasting, chanting, walking a labyrinth, and other religious practices have been used to align the body with the realm of the spiritual. Like scanning for radio signals, the body adjusts its focus to tune in to sacred vibrations. Many miraculous events have resulted from such practices, including the curing of illnesses. It might be more accurate to say that these rituals reminded the body of its role as the instrument of the divine.

Think back to a time when you felt strongly in tune with a higher spiritual realm, whether you refer to that realm as God or Goddess, your Source, nature, or some other name. What helped you tune in? Was it meditating, gardening, or praying? Did statues, sage, or fire invoke this state of intimate communion with the divine? Try to recall what you were doing that supported this closeness. If no particular spiritual practice prompted it, can you identify anything from that experience that you could now turn into a regular practice in order to induce this state of union routinely?

Spiritual transcendence can be achieved through simple activities such as gazing at a favorite painting on your wall or fingering a collection of smooth, colorful stones. Sitting on your porch looking at the sunset may help you suspend your sense of separation and arouse an all-absorbing knowing of being in union with all that is. Whether you use such simple entryways to the divine or exercise a disciplined practice such as yoga, fingering your beads, or chanting, build your daily schedule around this activity. Make a habit of fostering and maintaining your body-spirit connection through both intention and regular rituals and practices.

You can turn many of your ordinary daily activities into rituals of mindfulness. Thich Nhat Hanh teaches that doing the dishes can be a sacred act. Fully absorb yourself in washing each plate and cup as if it's the most important activity in the world for you to be doing at that moment. When you walk, walk mindfully—with your mind clear of unnecessary thoughts and your attention absorbed in the act of putting one foot after the other forward. The act of being *present* will bring you into the Presence. As Hanh says, "We do not have to die to enter the Kingdom of Heaven. In fact we have to be fully alive . . . . When we take one conscious breath, aware of our eyes, our heart, our liver, and our non-toothache, we are transported to Paradise right away."

Open up to love

Nothing can open up the channels to the divine more quickly than expressing love. Love is the very stuff of the divine. Some quantum physicists suggest that love is the energy that propels everything into being and keeps it active in an endless, dynamic flow. By recognizing that we are part of the energy field of love, and acting accordingly, we experience ourselves as one with all that is. In expressing our love (unconditional love, that is—with the well-being of others as our only goal), it's as if we pick up the energy current of universal love and let it flow through our body. We *become* loving. We might even say we *become love.*

Expressing love is a physical act. It begins with the heart. We open our heart to caring feelings that prompt us to want to give to others in some way. In fact, when we feel love in our heart, the electromagnetic energy of that feeling reaches out several feet from our body. We literally "touch" other people by generating feelings of love, compassion, appreciation, and other caring emotions. Already, we are love in action.

I remember a meeting I once had with a work colleague whose typically testy attitude made me very reluctant to talk with her. My task (given to me by my supervisor) was to instruct this colleague to change what she was doing on a project we has been assigned to do together. I anticipated a bristled response and felt quite anxious as she came into my office for the meeting. But I recalled the power of generating love in my heart and took a brief moment to call up a feeling of love and appreciation for this woman. I felt what I would describe as a rush of the divine pulsing through my heart, and my attitude toward her changed. As I delivered my instructions, I felt genuine care for her, and talking with her seemed easy. Because of my loving disposition, I felt *at one* with her, and I was able to approach my task with an appreciation for her needs and point of view. The conversation went smoothly, and she agreed to do the new procedures.

Women are prone to be loving and giving. We tend to be caretakers for everyone around us. By midlife, we've had a lot of practice at expressing love. It's a joy to be around women who seem naturally to exude a deep caring for others, and it's a joy to give to others in this naturally loving way.

For some women, though, their identity is tied up in doing for others. Their giving results in part from a genuine care for others, but mixed in with that caring is a need to be valued. Giving assures them that they have something worthwhile to offer, that they *count.* Marlene, the woman in chapter 7 who felt she had to be giving all the time, is a good example of someone caught up in such approval-seeking rescue missions. In one way, she felt good when she helped someone out, but at the same time, her giving had an element of desperation to it. If she couldn't jump in and give, she felt unworthy or *guilty.* Women such as Marlene are also hesitant to receive from others. When someone offers them help, that only proves to them that they're not good enough, that they've failed at having something to give instead. In seeking good-girl approval to fill their empty cup of worthiness, they block out what they truly long for—unconditional love. They can neither give it nor receive it easily.

This distinction is important. Being loving is not a performance to be approved (internally or externally) or a competitive sport at which to excel. We don't have to do certain things to be loving. Rather, an act of love starts and ends with a deep knowing of our worthiness—claiming our oneness with the divine stuff of love. When we know without question that the divine flame of love burns in us, we act not out of moral goodness but with a fire that can't help but spread. Whether love is flowing to us or from us, then, is all the same. Giving and receiving are hardly two separate acts. As we make ourselves at home with our loving nature, they are both present all the time.

Your body can clue you in to the distinction between good-girl kindness and confident, boundless loving. The next time you feel "obligated" to give your time, money, or a gift, notice how your body responds. Does your jaw tighten slightly? Do your teeth clench? Do your toes wriggle? Does your chest sink? Pay attention to where you feel contracted. A sense of obligation immediately creates some kind of internal conflict between your desire to be "acceptable"—to meet someone's expectations—and your preferences for how you use your time and money. If a sense of obligation alone drives your giving, your body will tend to tighten and pull inward.

By contrast, note your body's state when you're asked to give and your response is coming from a deep sense of love and caring. Is your posture upright? Are your facial muscles relaxed? Do you feel full of energy? You will probably notice a general feeling of expansiveness. Your arms may stretch open, ready to both give and receive. Even if you choose to say no to the request, your voice and mannerisms will exude confidence and kindness.

In which state do you think you are more closely in touch with your spiritual realm? Unless the "obligation" giving becomes steeped in genuine love, your body will continue to reflect a state of spiritual dissonance. Of course, I'm not suggesting you should avoid giving when a sacrifice on your part is what's needed. You may be the only one available to bathe a combative and unappreciative parent who can no longer care for herself. To do so means you may indeed need to make sacrifices. The word *sacrifice*, however, does not mean to strain yourself or give up something. It comes from Latin words that mean to "make holy."

How can difficult and distasteful chores be made holy? By immersing yourself in the practices talked about in this chapter, especially mindfulness and unconditional love. Even cleaning someone's messy bottom can become a holy act when it is done with mindful reverence. When giving and receiving are seen as one continual circle of love, then whatever we receive at any moment, even the smell of garbage, can be seen as a gift.

When in harmony with the divine, we love whatever comes our way. Gratitude and compassion are natural outgrowths of this love. While cleaning up litter during a walk in the park, I can be grateful—for my ability to bend over and pick up things, for my sense of beauty, and for those who have taught me its importance. I can feel compassion for the litterers for the sickness they have that leaves them immune to the damage they're doing. I can remember and feel compassion for myself for all the times I've been insensitive and inconsiderate. All these responses reflect very practically how, in the ordinariness of everyday life, our physical and spiritual dimensions can live in harmony.

Let your inner artist loose

All major spiritual traditions have used music to unite body and spirit. Chanting, hymn-singing, drumming, keening, and orchestral music are among the ways we physically tune ourselves to divine vibrations. From ancient times, believers in the spirit world have sketched, painted, and sculpted to express the mysteries of the divine. People of many cultures have danced in circles, in trances, in ritualized and creative forms, swirling into states of what I like to call transcen*dance*, a word coined by Joan Erikson. The theatre stage has hosted stories of deities from ancient lands and contemporary saints. Other art forms using cameras and computers have offered newer means of expressing spiritual themes creatively. Clearly, the arts have the ability to induce communion with the divine.

One of the activities I have participated in is a type of circle dancing called Dances of Universal Peace. These dances involve simple dance steps and gestures repeated many times, sometimes with partners. The movements are mostly done slowly and reverently, while the dancers sing repeatedly a short saying or a verse from a spiritual song. Songs are included from a wide range of faith traditions. The repetitive nature of the songs and movements creates a meditative state through a quieting of the mind, a rhythmic flow for the body, and the prayerful, melodic sounds. Body, mind, and spirit all seem to feel at home in this peaceful dance form.

In retreat settings and workshops, I invite women into creative dancing to express the divine spirit moving through them. Some women feel a little intimidated at first, fearful that they don't know how to create their own dance or that someone is watching them with a critical eye. But movement that arises from the inner promptings of Spirit can never be *wrong*. Rather, it is freeing. And it's beautiful, whatever form it takes. The human body is made to express the divine Spirit, and creative dance gives women permission to express it with fullness and grace.

As I provide guidance for the dancing, one of the processes I use is called *mesmerization*. I ask the women to find one thing in the room on which to focus their undivided attention—a plant, a wall feature, a glass of water. They then dance in response to whatever has caught their eye. The dance becomes a meditative exercise. Their attention is wrapped mindfully around one central point, which "mesmerizes" them. Like using a mantra in sitting meditation, this pointed attention frees them from distraction and allows them to explore with concentrated receptivity whatever has called to them in the room.

In some spiritual belief systems, any one thing in the universe is thought to contain the entire universe. Eric Butterworth, in *The Creative Life,* says it this way: "God cannot be more present anywhere than he is present everywhere." In other words, if you grasp and deeply engage with the essence of any one thing, you're engaged with everything—you're in union with the All. It's much like when you first fall deeply in love. Suddenly, because you love one person so intently, everyone and everything seems beautiful, and you fall in love with the whole world. The mesmerization dance has a similar effect. It engages the women in "loving" one thing intently by giving it their full attention and letting it evoke a creative response in them. The dancing, as it were, sweeps that love wide to take in all things.

Recall a moment in your life when a song, a dance, or some other artistic experience mesmerized you, lifting you beyond the realm of the ordinary. Re-enter this experience as fully as you can through Active Reminiscing, as described in chapter 12. What are you doing physically? Who or what has inspired your activity? How does your body feel compared to its ordinary state? In what ways is a sense of the divine registering in your body?

In order to keep alive your artistic link to Spirit, expose yourself often to the work of visual and performing artists who inspire you. Engage in artistic creativity of your own. Use the ideas from this chapter to help you get started discovering and expressing your spirituality through the arts. Live the life of the Creator.

What Does Your Body Have to Say?

OBSERVE AND REFLECT

IN SYNC WITH THE DIVINE: Review your life and make note of the times in your life when you felt most in sync with the divine. What was happening at these times? What was your source of inspiration? How did your body feel? Look for ways to re-create now the circumstances and inspiration from these times in a way that will reawaken or deepen your awareness of your body-mind-spirit union.

BEYOND "OBLIGATION": Make a list of the "obligations" you have in your life. Notice your body state as you get in touch with this sense of obligation about each of these items. Gently release all expectations of yourself and others. Instead, see yourself as filled with all the love in the universe. Imagine having within you everything you need to serve others without strain in a loving, appreciative, and compassionate way. Immerse yourself in this belief, generating the associated feelings in your heart and in every cell of your body. Know and experience your oneness with the all-present, all-loving divine Spirit. Let any sense of your unworthiness drop into the ocean of universal love and dissolve. Stay with this process until you feel the stress in your body lower and a peaceful state of mind emerge. Then, with your body and mind reflecting this loving spirit-based identity, decide which services on your list you're willing and able to offer freely and joyfully. Take the others off your to-do list. Thank your body and spirit for helping you in this discovery process.

WRITE

REWRITE THE BODY-SPIRIT SPLIT STORY: Write the story of how you learned to separate body and spirit as you grew up, if you did. Then rewrite the story, emphasizing the union of body, mind, and spirit.

LIVE

MESMERIZATION: Find a painting, sculpture, or other spiritual image that inspires you. Also choose music that is uplifting. With the music playing, gaze intently at the image you've chosen, allowing yourself to be mesmerized by it. Open yourself to respond creatively. Let it lead you to pray or meditate in a new way, create and sing a song or chant, dance freely, draw or paint. Use this activity anytime you feel your contact with the divine growing a little stale.

SPIRITUAL SUPPORT IN COMMUNITY: Participate in religious services, chanting or drumming groups, or women's spiritual circles that support your consciousness of your body-mind-spirit union.

Before You're Done

Old age has been given a bad name. It has its downside, to be sure. But an old body is not a dead body. Even if illness or certain losses limit us in some ways as the years pass, our body is still very much alive and capable in other ways. Yet too many older people sit glued to their chairs as if waiting for their graves to open up and suck them in. I sometimes see this when I visit people who are in their sixties and older, whether they're living in retirement or assisted-living communities or on their own. The feared image many of us have of old age—being slumped in a chair, staring at the TV, falling asleep, or playing endless bingo—is all too prevalent in reality. What a waste!

Unless you begin to appreciate and capitalize on the marvels of your body in midlife, that could be your destiny. Begin now to create the kind of old age you want for yourself. Imagine your body remaining vibrant and healthy until the end, and live each day as if it knows no bounds. No matter your age or condition, your body can be an ongoing resource for learning, pleasure, and creative expression.

In a Free Motion session I led at a senior-living campus, a woman who looked to be in her mid-seventies showed up in a wheelchair, with braces holding up her back and her neck erect. A fall had damaged Mary's body but not her spirit.

Declaring that her pain level "on a scale of one to ten is twenty," Mary still wanted to take part in the dancing. And she did. With a wide smile and all the energy she could muster, she stretched and lifted and waved her arms gaily to the music. Eileen, who had suffered a stroke and whose walk was wobbly, came to dance, too. Whether on her feet with a partner helping her remain upright or seated in a chair with her arms and legs in motion, she entered into the fun of it all. Even when Mary chided her for not using a cane to keep from falling, Eileen, whom I guessed to be past eighty, rebuffed Mary's caution, saying, "People are always telling me that, but even though my wings are clipped, I'm going to let myself fly."

Women like these give me hope.

Chapter Notes

Chapter 1

p. 5: Quote from Thomas Moore, *Care of the Soul.* New York: Harper Perennial, 1992, p. 155.

p. 5: Quotes from Judith Blackstone, audiotape "Subtle Self Work." Woodstock, NY: Realization Center.

p. 6: Quote from Eckhart Tolle, *A New Earth: Awakening to Your Life's Purpose.* New York: Penguin, 2005, p. 250.

p. 11: The "My Hands" poem exercise was developed by Elders Share the Arts in New York City. Contact information: Elders Share the Arts, Inc. 138 South Oxford Street, Brooklyn, NY 11217. Phone: (718) 398-3870. This poem exercise and other exercises for helping older people create "Living History Theatre" from their memories are described by Susan Perlstein, founder of Elders Share the Arts and Executive Director of the National Center for Creative Aging, in *A Stage for Memory: A Guide to the Living History Theatre Program of Elders Share the Arts.* Brooklyn, NY: The National Center for Creative Aging, 2004.

Chapter 2

p. 15: Quote from Edith Mucke, *The 85th Year.* St. Cloud, MN: North Star Press of St. Cloud, 2001, p. 12.

p. 20: Masaru Emoto's work with water crystals is discussed in his book *The Hidden Messages in Water.* New York: Atria Books, 2005.

p. 20: Scientists at the Institute of HeartMath in Boulder Creek, California have studied the intelligence of the heart and created the Freeze-Frame® technique and other processes for reducing stress and improving overall health. These processes and the research done on them are described by Howard Martin and Doc Childre in *The HeartMath Solution* (San Francisco: HarperSanFrancisco, 1999) and in other books written by the Institute's staff, as well as at www.heartmath.org.

p. 21: Quote from Myrtle Fillmore, *Myrtle Fillmore's Healing Letters.* Unity Village, MO: Unity Books, 1981, p. 21.

Chapter 4

p. 48: Sheila Rubin, LMFT, RDT/BCT, leads Life Stories Self-Revelatory Performance Drama Therapy Workshops in Berkeley, California. Her work is featured at www.thehealingstory.com.

p. 51: Focusing, developed by Eugene T. Gendlin, is a self-discovery and healing process based on body awareness. It is used widely by psychotherapists. Basic instructions for focusing are given at www.focusing.org and in Gendlin's book *Focusing.* New York: Everest House, 1978.

Chapter 5

p. 60: The work of Albert Pesso is quite remarkable. Now in his eighties, Pesso continues to speak to public and professional audiences and to train therapists in PBSP throughout the world. Information about the PBSP process and Pesso's calendar can be found at www.pbsp.com.

Quoted passages from Maggie Scarf, beyond my personal interview with her, are taken from her book *Secrets, Lies, Betrayals: How the Body Holds the Secrets of a Life, and How to Unlock Them.* New York: Ballantine, 2005.

p. 60: "leave their symptomatic calling cards," p. 5.

p. 61: "summoning up a person's feelings, emotions, and sensations," p. 253.

p. 61: "a taste of *what it would be like* to have had a different, more benign past and thus . . . engender[s] more hope-filled expectations . . . that are rooted in the body," p. 254.

p. 63: "It is for this reason that children who've been severely stressed during their earliest years will so often grow up to become adults who are deaf to their own bodily cues and warning signals," p. 101.

p. 64: "Her inner state is one of high arousal, and she is highly likely to respond in exaggerated ways to all sorts of minor challenges. Thus, a passing criticism from a boss, friend, or lover can precipitate the classic bodily reactions to a situation of crisis: a speeded-up heartbeat; clenched chest muscles; shallow, rapid breathing; and an outpouring of crisis situation neurohormones. Although outwardly the person may appear to be responding calmly, her body is in a state of perennial readiness to meet with threat, and perfectly ordinary, neutral kinds of events can be experienced as catastrophic ordeals," p. 102.

Chapter 6

Quotes from Arnold Mindell, PhD, are taken from *The Quantum Mind and Healing: How to Listen and Respond to Your Body's Symptoms.* Charlottesville, VA: Hampton Roads, 2004.

p. 82: "You are having big dreams in your body and (in a way) are lucky to receive dramatic messages from the force of silence," p. 16.

p. 83: "apparently unanswerable questions meant to increase our consciousness," p. 5.

p. 83: "Your symptoms of fatigue and persistent aches and chest pressure are the beginnings of a dance. Let your body dance and express whatever is in your chest creating that pressure," p. 21.

Quotes from Eckhart Tolle are taken from two sources:

p. 83: [Negative emotions leave] "a residue of emotional pain, which is stored in the cells of the body." Kathy Juline, "Awakening to Your Life's Purpose: An Interview with Eckhart Tolle," *Science of Mind,* October 2006, p. 20.

The following quotes from Eckhart Tolle are taken from his book *The Power of Now.* Novato, CA: New World Library, 1999:

p. 83 "In a fully functional organism . . . an emotion has a very short life span." [However,] "when you are not in your body, an emotion can survive inside you for days or weeks, or join with other emotions of a similar frequency that have merged and become the pain-body, a parasite that can live inside you for years, feed on your energy, lead to physical illness, and make your life miserable," p. 100.

p. 84: "inner body" or "subtle energy field that pervades the entire body and gives vibrant life to every organ and every cell," p. 93.

Quotes from Myrtle Fillmore are taken from *Myrtle Fillmore's Healing Letters.* Unity Village, MO: Unity Books, 1981.

p. 85: "emaciated little woman," p. 16.

p. 85: "In seeking health, we are to pray for an understanding of our oneness with God, to claim it," p. 105.

p. 85: "lost track of our hold on the gifts of God," p. 104.

p. 85: "our body temple is the fruit of our mind," p. 78.

p. 86: "looks into all his thought habits to see that they are prompted by faith and divine love and wisdom and life and joy and freedom," p. 108.

p. 86: "acquaints himself with the different parts of the body, and learns what it is they are truly built for. He learns what each needs and supplies them," p. 108.

Chapter 8

Quotes from Joan Erikson are taken from Joan Anderson's book *A Walk on the Beach: Tales of Wisdom from an Unconventional Woman.* New York: Broadway Books, 2005.

p. 110: "We're taught early on to stop sensing the world. Parents say no to their toddlers all the time, when all their child wants to do is to sense the word around him. Pity, isn't it! Overdose on the sense is what I say, all the way through life," p. 62.

p. 110: "We all need to unlearn the rules that are set up for us by others," p. 26.

p. 110: "Make time to play each day . . . We're asses if we don't," p. 217.

p. 111: "Look, there isn't anything that I do that I don't enjoy. If I do it then I enjoy it. But playful activities are the best because they are goalless, the result is unknown, and they are full of fantasy, imagination, and random discovery. What can beat that?" p. 217.

Chapter 10

p. 124: The work of Anthony Hyatt with Quicksilver is part of Arts for the Aging, a program in Bethesda, Maryland that regularly sends artists into local senior day care centers and nursing homes to engage the people there in artistic activities. Visit www.aftaarts.org to learn more.

p. 124: Kairos Dance Theatre is an intergenerational dance company in Minneapolis, led by artistic director Maria Genné. The Kairos performing company includes dancers from preschool age to people in the nineties and has performed at many local and national events. The company also regularly works with frail older adults, including those with Alzheimer's. Their website is www.kairosdance.org.

p. 125: The quote from Pearls of Wisdom member Amatullah Saleem appears on http://arts.endow.gov/resources/Accessibility/aa/conversations.html, as part of a series of profiles of older adults prepared in conjunction with 2005 Mini-Conference on Creativity and Aging in America.

p. 125: Senior theatres are popping up all over the country. The Senior Theatre Resource Center and ArtAge Publications, based in Portland, Oregon, offer many resources for senior theatres. Learn about them at www.seniortheatre.com.

p. 128: The landmark study directed by Dr. Gene Cohen, Director of the Center for Aging, Health and Humanities at George Washington University, has shown the positive health impact (physical, mental, and social) of participation by older adults in the creative arts. The 2001 study, called "The Creativity and Aging Study: The Impact of Professionally Conducted Cultural Programs on Older Adults," was sponsored by the National Endowment for the Arts, the National Institute of Mental Health, AARP, and others. Dr. Cohen studied three weekly programs conducted by professional artists—a senior choir in Washington, D.C.; a visual arts project in San Francisco; and a multidisciplinary program in New York City. Participants, with an average age of eighty, fared better on several critical health measures compared to their counterparts in control groups at each location.

Chapter 11

pp. 168–169: I found "On Turning 45" on a website called "Women's Journeys," which contains wonderful writings by women on many personal topics. Annie Kemp's essay appears at www.womensjourneys.com/html/love_turning45.html. Kemp graciously allowed me to reprint it in this book.

Chapter 13

p. 175: Quote from Thich Nhat Hanh is from *Touching Peace: Practicing the Art of Mindful Living*. Berkeley: Parallax Press, 1992, p. 8.

p. 178: I found Joan Erikson's use of the word *transcendance* in Joan Anderson's *A Walk on the Beach*.

p. 179: The Dances of Universal Peace were originated by Samuel L. Lewis in California in the 1960s and have since become a global movement. They are offered in schools, religious institutions, health centers, prisons, and other settings. Learn more about them at www.dancesofuniversalpeace.org.

p. 179: Quote from Eric Butterworth is taken from his book *The Creative Life*. New York: Tarcher/Putnam, 2001, p. 130.

Bibliography

Anderson, Joan. *A Walk on the Beach: Tales of Wisdom from an Unconventional Woman.* New York: Broadway Books, 2005.

Blackstone, Judith. *The Subtle Self: Personal Growth and Spiritual Practice.* Berkeley, CA: North Atlantic Books, 1991.

Butterworth, Eric. *The Creative Life.* New York: Tarcher/Putnam, 2001.

Childre, Doc, and Howard Martin. *The HeartMath Solution: The Institute of HeartMath's Revolutionary Program for Engaging the Power of the Heart's Intelligence.* San Francisco: HarperSanFrancisco, 2000.

Cohen, Gene D. *The Creative Age: Awakening Human Potential in the Second Half of Life.* New York: HarperCollins, 2001.

Emoto, Masaru. *The Hidden Messages in Water.* New York: Atria Books, 2005.

Fillmore, Myrtle. *Myrtle Fillmore's Healing Letters.* Unity Village, MO: Unity, 1981.

Gendlin, Eugene T. *Focusing.* New York: Everest House, 1978.

Goldman, Connie. *Late-Life Love: Romance and New Relationships in Later Years.* Minneapolis, MN: Fairview Press, 2006.

Hanh, Thich Nhat. *Touching Peace: Practicing the Art of Mindful Living.* Berkeley, CA: Parallax Press, 1992.

Hillman, James. *The Force of Character and the Lasting Life.* New York: Random House, 1999.

Keen, Sam. *Learning to Fly.* New York: Broadway Books, 1999.

Knaster, Mirka. *Discover the Body's Wisdom.* New York: Bantam, 1996.

Mindell, Arnold. *The Quantum Mind and Healing: How to Listen and Respond to Your Body's Symptoms.* Charlottesville, VA: Hampton Roads, 2004.

Moore, Thomas. *Care of the Soul.* New York: HarperPerennial, 1992.

Mucke, Edith. *The 85th Year.* St. Cloud, MN: North Star Press of St. Cloud, 2001.

Plonka, Lavinia. *What Are You Afraid Of?* New York: Tarcher/Penguin, 2004.

Scarf, Maggie. *Secrets, Lies, Betrayals.* New York: Random House, 2004.

Tolle, Eckhart. *A New Earth: Awakening to Your Life's Purpose.* New York: Penguin, 2005.

———. *The Power of Now.* Novato, CA: New World Library, 1999.

Wuthrow, Robert. *Creative Spirituality: The Way of the Artist.* Berkeley, CA: University of California Press, 2001.

Helpful Websites

www.creativeaging.org Provides information from the National Center for Creative Aging on artists throughout the nation who engage older adults in the arts. This website also offers other resources on arts and aging.

www.essential-motion.com Features information about Karen Roeper's work on personal transformation through movement and body awareness.

www.feldenkrais.com The Feldenkrais Educational Foundation of North America provides information about the Feldenkrais Method and local practitioners.

www.groupmotion.org Provides information on the Philadelphia-based Group Motion Dance Company, which offers weekly improvisational dance opportunities as well as weeklong retreats for the public.

www.hakomiinstitute.com Offers information on Hakomi mind/body therapy and provides a directory of practitioners.

www.heartmath.org and **www.heartmath.com** Describes the Institute of HeartMath's research and resources that shed light on the power of the heart and show how to access it for less stress and better health.

www.nadt.org A resource for finding local drama therapists and information about training as a drama therapist.

www.pbsp.com Provides information on Pesso Boyden System Psychomotor (PBSP), a comprehensive therapeutic approach to trauma healing that involves creating alternate virtual memories in the mind and body.

www.realizationcenter.com Offers information on the Subtle Self work of Judith Blackstone, which teaches attunement to fundamental consciousness through the body.

www.selfacceptance.us Describes the work of Cherie McCoy, whose Self Acceptance Training guides people to self-discovery and a deep level of self-acceptance.

www.thirdage.com Provides resources on later life, including a blog featuring commentary by leading authors on Third Age topics.

www.womensjourneys.com A friendly site edited by Rochelle Jourdan, featuring essays and articles by women about issues that matter to women.

The "Appreciate Your Body" CD by Pat Samples, which contains guided instructions for the Conscious Body Awareness exercise on page 7 and the Body Appreciation exercise on page 22, is available from www.patsamples .com.

Exercise Index